AMERICAN NURSES ASSOCIATION
CENTER FOR CONTINUING EDUCATION AND PROFESSIONA
Required Disclosures to Participants

W9-BPM-836

Successful Completion of this Continuing Nursing Education (CNE) Activity:

In order to receive full contact hour credit for this CNE activity, you must:
- Be registered for this activity and pay required fees,
- Be present no later than five (5) minutes after starting time,
- Participate in individual or group activities, such as discussion, exercises, practice questions, pre-/post-testing, etc.
- Remain until the scheduled ending time
- Complete the online CNE survey.

Up to **14 contact hours** (60 minute contact hour) will be awarded for successful completion of this CNE activity. Partial credit may be awarded based on each session attended

Please ensure that your email is accurate on the roster/sign in sheet. An evaluation link will be emailed to you to access the online evaluation survey and verification of attendance. The demographic information will not be tied to your evaluation report. This is for the CE records.

The survey will be emailed to you and remain open for four (4) weeks following the workshop or webinar. You must complete the online survey and verification of attendance before it closes in order to earn contact hours for this activity.

- Please note that the agenda in your program materials identify the activity purpose/goal(s), session times, objectives, content outline, presenters, and teaching-learning strategies. The sessions, objectives, and presenters on the agenda correspond with the evaluation.

- You will be able to download your "certificate of completion" after completing the evaluation. Partial certificates may be downloaded in some cases or an adjusted certificate will be emailed to you four (4) weeks after the evaluation survey closes.

If you do not meet the four (4) week deadline for completing the online survey and verification of attendance, you may contact the American Nurses Association to receive your certificate for an additional fee as follows.

> Send your written request and check or money order made payable to the American Nurses Association in the sum of $20.00 per certificate to:
> American Nurses Association
> P O Box 504410
> St. Louis, MO   63150-4410
> Include your name, address and e-mail address. Certificate(s) will be e-mailed to the address provided.
> If you attended a conference or seminar with multiple sessions you must identify each session you attended by title in your request.
> Allow 4-6 weeks for processing.

Here is the link to contact ANCC: Livesemr@ana.org

Psychiatric-Mental Health Nursing Review Course Agenda
Contact Hours: 14.0 Learning Strategies: Lecture, Slides, Discussion, Q & A

Gap in Knowledge: The need for knowledge of current practice and review materials to prepare for the ANCC Psychiatric-Mental Health Nursing certification exam.

Purpose: To provide clinical nurses with current clinical practice information to be utilized in the care of psychiatric patients and to provide review materials for nurses desiring ANCC Psychiatric-Mental Health Nursing certification.

Timeframe	Session and Learning Objectives	Contact Hrs
	DAY ONE	
8:00 am - 9:45 am	**001: Neuroanatomy & Neurophysiology; The Nursing Process in Psychiatric Nursing: Assessment** **Learning Objectives:** 1. Review the major structures and functions of the brain and the impact on function and dysfunction. 2. Identify the assessment component focusing on data collection for optimal patient outcomes. 3. Discuss biopsychosocial (physical, emotional, growth and development) norms that promote optimal patient outcomes.	1.75
9:45 am - 10:00 am	**BREAK**	
10:00 am - 11:45 pm	**002: The Nursing Process in Psychiatric Nursing: Diagnosis & Planning (Part 1)** **Learning Objectives:** 1. Identify appropriate nursing diagnoses for improved patient outcomes. 2. Describe pathophysiological alterations and problems that compromise optimal patient outcomes.	1.75
11:45 pm - 12:45 pm	**LUNCH**	
12:45 pm - 3:00 pm	**003: The Nursing Process in Psychiatric Nursing: Diagnosis & Planning (Part 2)** **Learning Objectives:** 1. Discuss appropriate care plans utilizing evidence-based strategies and therapeutic environments for improved patient outcomes. 2. Identify nurse-initiated and collaborative (e.g., interprofessional) strategies for improved patient outcomes.	2.25
3:00 pm - 3:15 pm	**BREAK**	
3:15 pm - 4:30 pm	**004 : Pharmacological, Biological, & Integrative Therapies (Part 1)** **Learning Objectives:** 1. Discuss nurse-initiated and collaborative strategies related to the administration of psychotropic medications for improved patient outcomes. 2. Discuss the considerations for medication management of the psychiatric mental health population across the life span.	1.25

Psychiatric-Mental Health Nursing Review Course Agenda
Contact Hours: 14.0 Learning Strategies: Lecture, Slides, Discussion, Q & A

Timeframe	Session and Learning Objectives	Contact Hrs
	DAY TWO	
8:00 am - 9:30 am	**005: Pharmacological, Biological, & Integrative Therapies (Part 2)** **Learning Objectives:** 1. Discuss nurse-initiated and collaborative strategies related to the implementation of somatic, complementary and integrative treatments for improved patient outcomes. 2. Discuss the management of crises in guiding seclusion and restraint decisions.	1.5
9:30 am - 9:45 am	**BREAK**	
9:45 am - 11:30 am	**006: Nurse-Patient Relationships, Professional Development, & Leadership (Part 1)** **Learning Objectives:** 1. Discuss the role of the Registered Nurse (RN) in fostering and maintaining a therapeutic relationship with patients from differing cultural backgrounds. 2. Identify responsibilities and behaviors of the RN for professional development and accountability to self and the patient/family in complex health care settings.	1.75
11:30 am - 12:30 pm	**LUNCH**	
12:30 pm - 1:30 pm	**007: Nurse-Patient Relationships, Professional Development, & Leadership (Part 2)** **Learning Objectives:** 1. Identify RN roles that demonstrate leadership and professional accountability. 2. Discuss the importance of contributing to quality improvement in health systems.	1.0
1:30 pm - 2:45 pm	**008: Patient Education and Population Health** **Learning Objectives:** 1. Identify appropriate strategies for teaching-learning success in patient education as it relates to population health. 2. Identify counseling and other individual and group psychoeducational approaches that support patient-centered, family mental health. 3. Discuss the roles of the RN in advocating for the psychiatric mental health patient population, including eliminating stigma, discrimination, and criminalization.	1.25
2:45 pm - 3:00 pm	**BREAK**	
3:00 pm - 4:00 pm	**008: Patient Education and Population Health (continued)**	1.0
4:00 pm - 4:30 pm	**Summary/Question & Answer** **Test Taking Strategies, Content Outline, Testing Environment**	0.5

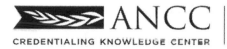

Psychiatric - Mental Health Nursing Review Course

Workshop

ANCC

Copyright Disclosure

Any recording or reproduction of materials associated with this review seminar is **NOT PERMITTED**, as this material is copyright-protected.

Thank you,

ANCC Institute Staff

© 2014 American Nurses Credentialing Center

ANCC

PREPARE WELL...
ANTICIPATE SUCCESS!

National Certified Nurses Day is March 19th

© 2014 American Nurses Credentialing Center

ANCC

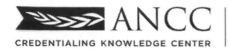

CATEGORY I: ASSESSMENT, DIAGNOSIS AND PLANNING

© 2014 American Nurses Credentialing Center

Session: 001
Neuroanatomy & Neurophysiology; The Nursing Process in Psychiatric Nursing: Assessment

---

001: Learning Objectives

1. Review the major structures and functions of the brain and the impact on function and dysfunction.
2. Identify the assessment component focusing on data collection for optimal patient outcomes.
3. Discuss biopsychosocial (physical, emotional, growth and development) norms that promote optimal patient outcomes.

© 2014 American Nurses Credentialing Center

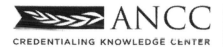
7

REVIEW: NEUROANATOMY AND NEUROPHYSIOLOGY

© 2014 American Nurses Credentialing Center

8

Functional Areas of the Cortex

- Different parts of the nervous system serve distinctly different functions
  - Motor- Precentral gyrus
  - Sensory- Postcentral gyrus
  - Visual area- Occipital cortex
  - Auditory area- Temporal cortex
  - Speech Broca's area in the inferior frontal gyrus
  - Receptive language- Wernicke's area in the posterior temporal cortex

© 2014 American Nurses Credentialing Center

9

Cortical Disruption (Dysfunction of Cortex)

- Dementia: Deterioration in intellectual and cognitive functions
  - Common signs and symptoms of deterioration:
    - Aphasia- Disruption of language function
    - Apraxia- Disturbance in the organization of voluntary action
    - Agnosia- Disorganization of perception and recognition
    - Amnesia- Dysfunction of memory processes
    - Alogia- Disruption of expressive language ability

© 2014 American Nurses Credentialing Center

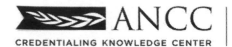
Divisions of the Nervous System

10

1. Central Nervous System (CNS): Most important in psychiatric disorders
   * Brain
   * Spinal Cord
2. Peripheral Nervous System (PNS): Connects CNS to receptors, muscles, and glands
   * Somatic Nervous System (NS): Connects CNS to skeletal muscles as in voluntary movement
   * Autonomic NS: Connects CNS to smooth muscle, cardiac muscle, glands as in visceral response
     1. Sympathetic Division: Stress activation
        * Fight, flight, fright, and sex
     2. Parasympathetic Division: Restoration and recovery
        * Digestion, growth, immune responses, and energy storage

© 2014 American Nurses Credentialing Center

Brain Subdivisions: Cerebrum and Brainstem

11

* Cerebrum: Two hemispheres joined by corpus callosum
  * Basal ganglia
  * Thalamus
  * Hypothalamus
  * Four Lobes
    1. Frontal
    2. Temporal
    3. Parietal
    4. Occipital

* Brainstem
  * Midbrain
  * Pons and Cerebellum
  * Medulla
  * Limbic System and Hippocampus
  * Reticular Formation

© 2014 American Nurses Credentialing Center

Basal Ganglia

12

* "Bundle of nerves" deep in the cerebrum.
* Critical role in motor function (movement) especially fine motor functioning.
  * Caudate (cravings originate here) and putamen, referred to as the "striatum," form the basal ganglia.
  * Nigrostriatal pathway is part of the extrapyramidal system (EPS), thus EPS medication side effects affect this area, one of which is movement.
* Bradykinesia, hyperkinesia, and hypokinesia all suggest disease of, or damage to, the basal ganglia!

© 2014 American Nurses Credentialing Center

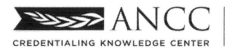

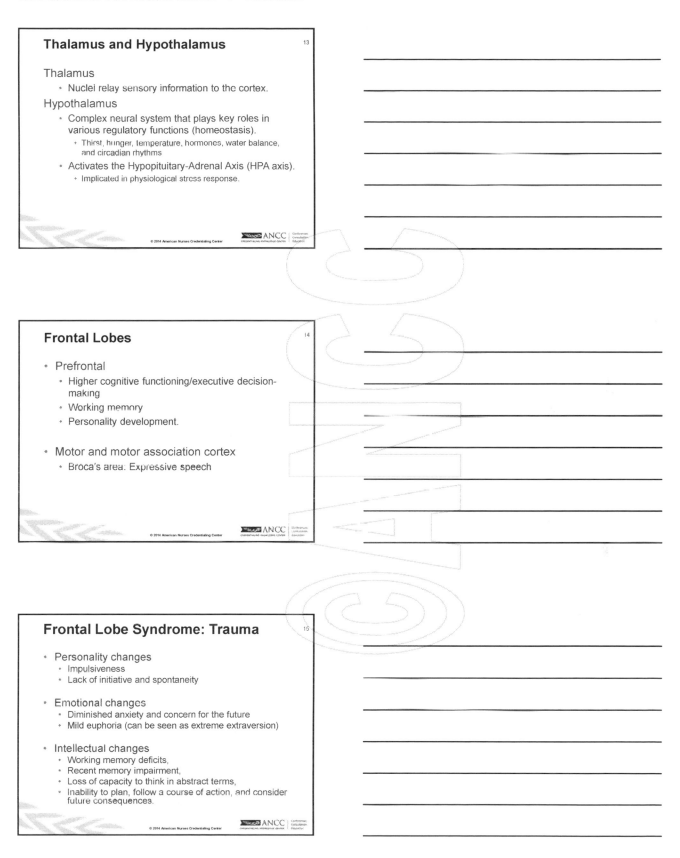

Thalamus and Hypothalamus

13

Thalamus
- Nuclei relay sensory information to the cortex.

Hypothalamus
- Complex neural system that plays key roles in various regulatory functions (homeostasis).
  - Thirst, hunger, temperature, hormones, water balance, and circadian rhythms
- Activates the Hypopituitary-Adrenal Axis (HPA axis).
  - Implicated in physiological stress response.

© 2014 American Nurses Credentialing Center

Frontal Lobes

14

- Prefrontal
  - Higher cognitive functioning/executive decision-making
  - Working memory
  - Personality development.

- Motor and motor association cortex
  - Broca's area. Expressive speech

© 2014 American Nurses Credentialing Center

Frontal Lobe Syndrome: Trauma

15

- Personality changes
  - Impulsiveness
  - Lack of initiative and spontaneity

- Emotional changes
  - Diminished anxiety and concern for the future
  - Mild euphoria (can be seen as extreme extraversion)

- Intellectual changes
  - Working memory deficits,
  - Recent memory impairment,
  - Loss of capacity to think in abstract terms,
  - Inability to plan, follow a course of action, and consider future consequences.

© 2014 American Nurses Credentialing Center

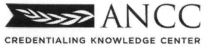
Temporal Lobes

16

- Hearing, Language, Learning, Memory, and Emotional Response.
  - Primary auditory (hearing) projection and association area
  - Wernicke's area: Receptive speech
  - Integrates visual experience with all forms of sensory information
  - Memory

Parietal Lobes

17

- Primary sensory cortex for visual spatial processing
- Association area integrates sensory input; main sensory receptive area for the sense of touch
- Processes discrete elements into meaningful wholes
- Cross-modal association and integration

Occipital Lobes

18

- Primary visual cortex
- Secondary sensory area
- Elaboration and synthesis of visual information
- Integration of visual and sensory information

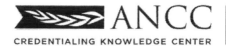

Brainstem

19

- Comprised of the:
  - Midbrain
  - Pons
  - Medulla
- Neurotransmitters, produced in the brainstem travel to diffuse brain areas, allowing for modulation of brain functions and are "excited" or "inhibited" by psychotropic medications.
- Neurotransmitter pathways are essential for modulating motor control, memory, mood, motivation, and metabolic states.

© 2014 American Nurses Credentialing Center

Cerebellum

20

- Movement, Balance, Posture
  - Gross movement control center
  - Maintains equilibrium and sense of balance
  - Calculates sequencing of muscle contractions
  - Deficits include ataxia (uncoordinated and inaccurate movements)
    - Romberg Test detects poor balance

© 2014 American Nurses Credentialing Center

Limbic System

21

- Limbic system functions:
  - Amygdala- Mediates mood, emotion, fear, and aggression
  - Hippocampus- Involved with memory
  - Prefrontal cortex
  - Cingulate gyrus
  - Mammillary bodies
  - Fornix

- Disorders of emotion, memory, and olfactory sense involve the limbic structures and their connections.

© 2014 American Nurses Credentialing Center

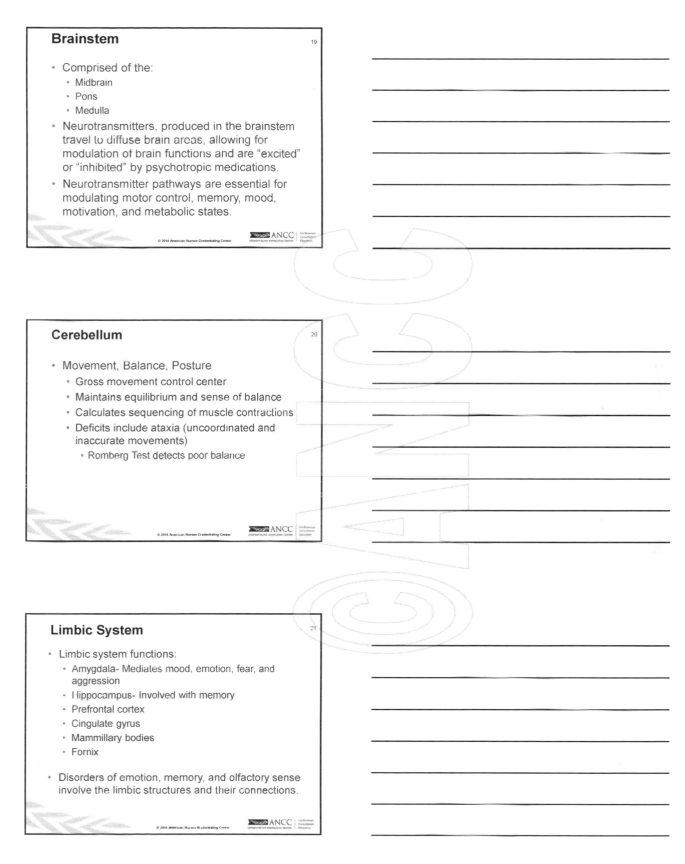

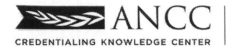
Neuron

22

- The brain "microprocessor"; information processor.
- Comprised of membrane, nucleus, cytoplasm, and organelles.
- Estimated 100 billion in the brain and in the heart and gut.
- Conducts impulses from one part of body to another.
- May receive input from 1 to 100,000 different axons.
- Three anatomically distinct regions
  - Cell body (soma)- Nucleus and cytoplasm,
  - Dendrites- Generally receive information, and
  - Axon: Generally sends information.

© 2014 American Nurses Credentialing Center

Glia (Glial) Cells

23

Three types:
1. Astrocytes- Provides nutrients to cells.
2. Oligodendrocytes- Forms myelin sheath around axons.
3. Microglia- Removes waste and debris.

Basic functions
- Supporting structures
- Guides migration of neurons during development
- Control extracellular concentrations of K+ and other ion

© 2014 American Nurses Credentialing Center

Synapse

24

- Area of space where a neuron electrically transfers chemical (neurotransmitter) information to another cell.

- The presynaptic cell area converts this electrical signal (action potential) to the postsynaptic cell, which "excite" or "inhibit" adjacent neurons.

http://www.nimh.nih.gov/health/educational-resources/brain-basics/nimh-brain-basics.pdf

© 2014 American Nurses Credentialing Center

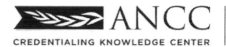
Neurotransmitters

25

- Are chemicals synthesized by neurons. They are
  - Present in presynaptic terminals,
  - Released at the terminal end via electrical activity,
  - Diffuses across synaptic cleft, and
  - Binds to specific receptors on the postsynaptic cell.

- Neuronal mechanisms
  - Diffusion
  - Enzymatic destruction: MAO's
  - Reuptake (pumped back into the neuron)

Major Neurotransmitter Categories

26

- Cholinergics
- Monoamines
- Amino acids
- Neuropeptides
- Cholinergic Type
  - Acetylcholine (AcH): Most common in CNS and PNS
    - Contraction and action of skeletal muscle, learning and memory, attention and arousal

---

Neurotransmitters and Functions

27

- Monoamine Types
  - Dopamine (DA or D_2)
    - Attention, executive functioning, motivation (reward and pleasure), addictions, mood, and movement
  - Norepinephrine (NE)
    - Arousal, concentration, learning and memory, mood, and stress response
  - Epinephrine (adrenaline) (E)
    - Stress response
  - Serotonin (5-HTP)
    - Mood, appetite, eating behavior, and sleep
  - Histamine
    - Involved in immune responses and allergies

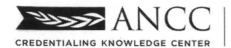
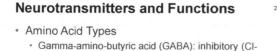

Neurotransmitters and Functions

28

- Amino Acid Types
  - Gamma-amino-butyric acid (GABA): inhibitory (Cl- into cell; K+ out of cell)
    - CNS depressant-like effects (acts like benzodiazepines, barbiturates, alcohol, other CNS depressants)
  - Glycine: Inhibitory
    - Motor and sensory information processing
  - Glutamate: Excitatory (Na+ and Ca+ into cell)
    - Most important for normal brain functioning
- Neuropeptides
  - Enkephalins, Endorphins, Substance P, Vasopressin, Insulin, Oxytocin, and Cholestokinin
    - Modulates pain and other biological function

© 2014 American Nurses Credentialing Center

New Fields of Study

29

Based on mind/body system integration
- Psychoneuroimmunology
- Psychoneuroendocrinology

NIMH 10-year project focused on mapping the brain (Based on a recent Presidential initiative started 2013.)
- BRAIN Initiative (BRAIN=Brain Research through Advancing Innovative Neurotechnology)

© 2014 American Nurses Credentialing Center

CATEGORY I A: ASSESSMENT

© 2014 American Nurses Credentialing Center

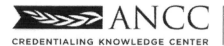

ANCC | Conferences. Consultation. Education.

CREDENTIALING KNOWLEDGE CENTER

Overview: Five Steps of the Nursing Process [31]

1. Assessment
   - Information collected and sources
2. Nursing Diagnosis
   - Problems seen, recognized, and known
3. Planning (Outcomes Identification)
   - Expectations derived from the goal setting
4. Implementation/Intervention
   - Clinical decisions made to improve patient condition
   - Actions: What nurse does?
5. Evaluation
   - How did clinical decisions/implementations work?

© 2014 American Nurses Credentialing Center

Assessment: What, Where, When, Who? [32]

- What is the problem?
- Where does the problem occur?
- When does the problem occur?
- Who or what makes the problem occur?
- What is the feared consequence related to the problem?

© 2014 American Nurses Credentialing Center

Assessment: Practice Standard 1 [33]

- RN collects and documents data/information related to patient's health history, medication regimen, and current health status. Assessment data is systematic and continuous.
- Corroborated/Obtained from multiple sources:
  - Patient,
  - Medical and pharmacy records,
  - EMT and law enforcement,
  - EAP referrals,
  - Collateral – Family, case workers, staff from previous facilities, significant others, teachers, and supervisors.

© 2014 American Nurses Credentialing Center

Assessment: Practice Standard 1

34

Components of medical and psychiatric history

- Physical examination:
  - Review of systems (ROS)
  - Vital signs and lab values
  - Radiologic studies (MRI, PET Scans, and CT Scans)
  - Allergies, medications: Effects, side effects, and reconciliation (list of all current medications)

- Psychosocial status
  - Mental status exam, other screens (i.e., depression, anxiety)
  - Substance use history (licit; illicit), alcohol, tobacco, other drug screens. *"How much…?"*
  - Motivation, coping responses
  - Reason for seeking health care
  - Strengths and weaknesses, general functioning
  - Ability to remain safe and refrain from harm (self/others)

© 2014 American Nurses Credentialing Center ANCC

Assessment: Practice Standard 1

35

- Components (continued)
  - Risk factors: Falls, pain, violence, aggression, suicidal ideation/homicidal ideation (SI/HI), genetics, deep vein thrombosis (DVT's), and sleep disorders (apnea, insomnia)
    - Family/ biographical information (genogram, history)
      - Relationships or roles
    - History of Abuse (physical, sexual, or emotional)
    - Sexual orientation
    - Gender identity
    - Vocational/occupational history
    - Spiritual, beliefs, and values
    - Developmental assessment
    - Congenital anomalies
    - Growth and development (milestones)

© 2014 American Nurses Credentialing Center ANCC

Neurological Basis of Development

36

- Developmental theories of Piaget, Freud, Erickson, etc. suggest neurological influences.
- Evidence: Caregiver reactions during first 2 years are internalized as distinct neural circuits, which may be modified through subsequent life experiences.
  - A pattern of terrifying experiences in infancy may flood the amygdala resulting in memory circuits that are hyperaroused.
  - Post-traumatic stress disorders represent over activity of the fear response.

© 2014 American Nurses Credentialing Center ANCC

Piaget's 4 Stages of Cognitive Development 37

1. From birth to age 2 : <u>Sensorimotor</u>
   * Sees the world through direct, physical action with people and things accessible through senses.
   * Progresses from motor and sensory reflexes to more deliberate/purposeful actions.
   * Begins the "schema" (i.e., knowledge) acquisition called object permanence, for example "peek-a-boo" games, which teaches that out-of-sight is not permanently gone (i.e., out of mind).
2. Age 2 to 7 : <u>Preoperational</u>
   * Symbols, images, words, and gestures can represent objects and events.
   * Imitates plays symbolically, uses graphic and mental imagery, language is egocentric, rigidity of thought, has semi-logical reasoning, and limited social cognition.

© 2014 American Nurses Credentialing Center ANCC

Piaget's 4 Stages of Cognitive Development (cont.) 38

3. Age 7 to 11 : <u>Concrete operations</u>
   * Knows that values remain the same (e.g., same volume or amount of water although appears different in different size containers, the volume is still the same).
     * Understands concept of conservation of quantity, weight, volume, length, and time based on reversibility by inversion or reciprocity.

4. Age 11 to Adolescence: <u>Formal operations</u>
   * Mental operations applied. Can classify, order, and reverse mental operations. Hypotheses can be generated, demonstrates abstract thinking abilities.

© 2014 American Nurses Credentialing Center ANCC

Freud's 5 Psychoanalytic Stages of Development 39

1. Oral (birth to 18 months)
   * Learns to handle anxiety through oral gratification
2. Anal (18 months to 3 years)
   * Learns independence and control with focus on excretory functions
3. Phallic (3 to 6 years)
   * Identifies with parent of same sex, starts to develop sexual identity

4. Latency (6 to 12 years)
   * Sexuality is repressed, focus is on relationships with same-sex peers
5. Genital (12 to adulthood)
   * Sexual interest (libido) is reawakened as secondary sex characteristics develop

© 2014 American Nurses Credentialing Center ANCC

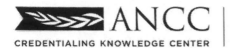

Basic Freudian Psychoanalytic Concepts

40

- All behavior has meaning.
- The unconscious plays an important role in understanding human behavior.
- Symptoms result from efforts to cope with anxiety and are related to unresolved developmental conflicts.
- Three parts to personality and development
  - Id is present at birth.
    - Serves to satisfy needs and immediate gratification
  - Ego begins to develop at 4 to 6 months.
    - Maintains contact with reality, which is the rationale part of personality
  - Superego begins to develop at about 3 to 6 years.
    - Serves as the conscience (i.e., a sense of right or wrong/morality)

© 2014 American Nurses Credentialing Center

Defense Mechanisms (Freudian)

41

Mostly unconscious, often inflexible coping patterns that protect one from an experience of stress and anxiety.

Interferes with:
- Rational decision-making and the ability to work productively.
- Reality-based ideation
- Interpersonal relationships.
- Moving forward beyond an impasse.

Repression	Denial
Suppression	Compensation
Dissociation	Rationalization
Identification	Reaction formation
Introjection	Displacement
Projection	Intellectualization
Splitting	Undoing
Regression	Sublimation

© 2014 American Nurses Credentialing Center

Erikson's 8 Stages of Man

42

Age	Developmental Conflict	Successful Resolution
Infant	Trust vs. mistrust	Drive and hope
Toddler	Autonomy vs. shame and doubt	Self-control and willpower
Preschool	Initiative vs. guilt	Direction and purpose
School Age	Industry vs. inferiority	Method and competence
Adolescence	Identity vs. role confusion	Devotion and fidelity
Young Adult	Intimacy vs. isolation	Affiliation and love
Adulthood	Generativity vs. stagnation	Production and care
Maturity	Ego integrity vs. despair	Renunciation and wisdom

© 2014 American Nurses Credentialing Center

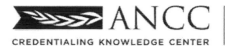

ANCC
CREDENTIALING KNOWLEDGE CENTER | Conferences. Consultation. Education.

Interpersonal Relationships: H.S. Sullivan's Psychodynamic Theory

43

- Anxiety is experienced interpersonally.
  - Behavior directed toward relief or prevention of anxiety.
  - Interpersonal security is feeling associated with relief of anxiety.
- Basic fear of rejection.
  - Importance of "significant other."
- Interpersonal relations within a social context influences personality development.
  - Perceptions of self result from reflected appraisals, for example "good-me, bad-me, not-me."

© 2014 American Nurses Credentialing Center ANCC

Kohlberg's Moral Development Theory

44

- Preconvention Period (2 to 12 years):
  - Stage 1: Obedience and punishment driven by ideas related to knowledge of consequences.
  - Stage 2: Self-interest behaviors determined by perceptions of what's best for self.
- Conventional Period (Adolescents and adults):
  - Stage 3: Interpersonal accord and conformity driven by social approval and disapproval.
  - Stage 4: Authority and social order driven by more universal understandings of right and wrong.
- Postconventional Period (Principled level):
  - Stage 5: Social contract driven-based on appreciating a more universal sense of general well-being for all.
  - Stage 6: Universal ethical principles moral "rightness" of a situation despite expectations and beliefs of others.

© 2014 American Nurses Credentialing Center ANCC

Examples of Standardized Assessment Tools Related to Mental Health Across the Life Span

45

- APGAR - For neonates
- DDST II - For infant/child
- HEADSS - For adolescents
- MSE: Child/Adult versions
- MMSE: Mini-Mental Status Exam
- Montreal Cognitive Assessment (MOCA)
- Suicide/Homicide (Lethality Assessment)
- AIMS: Abnormal Involuntary Movement Scale
- Pain Scale
- Intelligence Quotient (IQ)

- CAGE screening
- Hamilton Anxiety Scale
- Beck Depression Inventory
- Iowa Connors Rating Scale
- CIWA, Ar: Clinical Institute Withdrawal Assessment, Alcohol, revised (CIWA, Ar)
- COWS: Clinical Opioid Withdrawal Scale
- Clinical Institute Narcotic Assessment (CINA)
- Clinical Institute Withdrawal for Benzodiazepines (CIWA,B)
- Mini Nutritional Assessment (MNA)

© 2014 American Nurses Credentialing Center ANCC

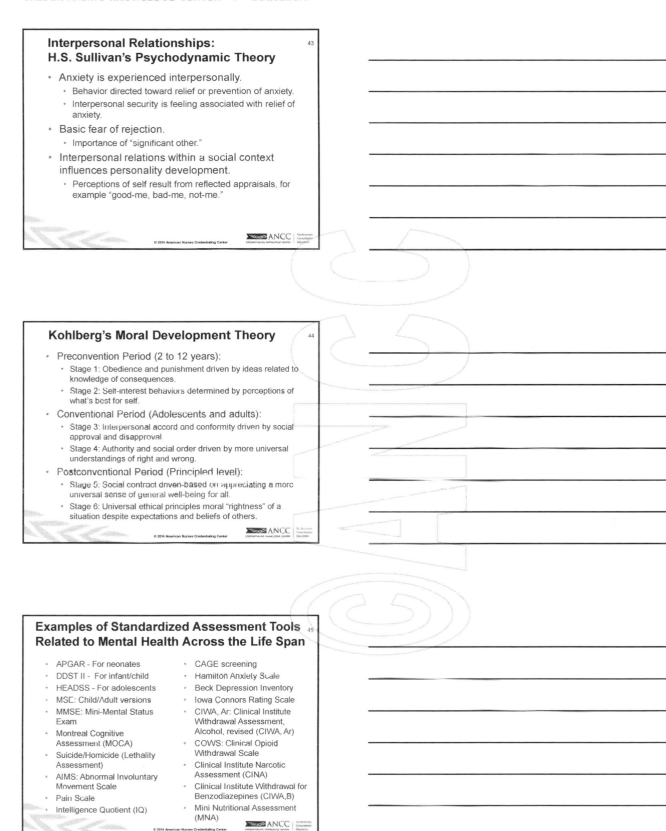

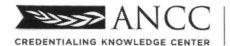
Examples of Standardized Assessment Tools 46
Related to Mental Health Across the Life Span

- Montgomery-Asberg Depression Rating Scale (MADRS)
- Columbia-Suicide Severity Rating Scale (C-CSSRS)
- Brief Psychiatric Rating Scale (BRPS)
- Young Mania Rating Scale (YMRS)
- McGowan Risk Assessment for Violence
- Fagerstrom Test for Nicotine Dependence

- Quality of Life Enjoyment and Satisfaction Questionnaire (Q-LES-Q-SF)
- Barnes Akathisia Rating Scale (BARS)
- Sheehan Disability Scale (SDS)
- Hamilton Rating Scale for Anxiety (HAM-A)
- PHQ-9: Patient Heath Questionnaire
- Yale-Brown OCD Scale
- PANSS: Positive and Negative Syndrome Scale

© 2014 American Nurses Credentialing Center   ANCC

Risk Factors for Childhood Disorders 47

- Early symptoms may manifest as problems with language skill development, communication (may be delayed), stereotypical gestures, play difficulties, enuresis, encopresis, and evidence of perceptual or sensory abnormalities.
- Disorders can be diagnosed as early as age 2.
  - Full range of symptoms may not be present until age 3 or later.
- Paucity (lack) of good screening tools for early diagnosis.
- Early diagnosis can lead to early interventions.

© 2014 American Nurses Credentialing Center   ANCC

Assessment: Neonate 48

- Optimal organogenesis emanates initially from the overall health and union of the sperm and ovum at conception.
- Maternal drug abuse (e.g., fetal alcohol syndrome), risky sexual behaviors (congenital HIV), and TORCH infections predispose risks for neurodevelopmental disabilities or intellectual disabilities:
  - Toxoplasmosis
  - Syphilis
  - Rubella
  - Cytomegalovirus (CMV)
  - Herpes Simplex Virus (HSV)

© 2014 American Nurses Credentialing Center   ANCC

Assessment: Neonate (Cont.)

49

- Birth weight averages 7 pounds head approximately 1/3 size of entire body.
- APGAR:
  - 0-10 rating scale of neonate conducted 1 and 5 minutes in postnatal period assigns score based on heart rate, respiratory effort, muscle tone, reflexes, color, irritability.
  - Score less than 3 = Problem

Assessment: Infant and Child

50

- Denver Developmental Screening Tool II (DDST-II) measurements in four areas
  1. Fine and gross motor abilities,
  2. Language,
  3. Personal and social abilities, and
  4. Adaptive abilities: Reach for specific objects.

Developmental Assessment: Sensory, Motor, Emotional, Language Milestones

51

- Development progresses from global to more specific
- Newborns
  - Can express pleasure.
- 2 weeks
  - Prefers mother's voice.
  - Can discriminate colors, smells, and tastes.
- 4 to 6 weeks
  - Whole face smiles and laughter.
- 4 months
  - Can balance head.
- 6 months
  - Can sit.

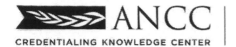

Developmental Assessment: Sensory, Motor, Emotional, Language Milestones

52

- 8 months
  - Has stranger anxiety.
- 10 months
  - Can creep, be pulled to feet, and have a crude prehensile grasp.
- 12 months
  - Can walk with help and grasp a small pellet.

© 2014 American Nurses Credentialing Center

Developmental Assessment: Sensory, Motor, Emotional, Language Milestones

53

Age 1
- Speaks in one-word sentences – "cookie."

Age 2
- Speaks in two-word sentences – "want cookie."
- Can run with ease, but not great skill.
- Can copy a circle.
- Displays anger when autonomy is threatened; guilt and remorse (moral development).

Age 3
- Can stand on one foot, dance, jump, and build a tower of 10 cubes.
- Can copy a cross.
- Attempts to control emotions.

© 2014 American Nurses Credentialing Center

Developmental Assessment: Sensory, Motor, Emotional, Language Milestones

54

Age 2-4
- Vocabulary increases rapidly.

Age 5
- Can skip and copy a square.

Age 6
- Can ride a bike with automatic ease.

© 2014 American Nurses Credentialing Center

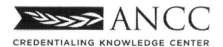
HEADSS Assessment

55

- Home and environment
- Education and Employment
- Eating
- Activities
- Drugs
- Sexuality
- Suicide/Depression

Assessment: Mental Status

56

- An ongoing patient-centered practice of the professional RN in all clinical settings.

- Acute changes lead to initiation of an emergent medical work-up and labs to diagnose and treat underlying medical conditions.

- Essential responsibilities
  - Maintain safety,
  - Monitor vital signs, and
  - Adequate nutritional status.

Mental Status Assessment

57

- Mental Status Exam (MSE)
  - An objective report of the patient's current mental state as observed by the nurse.

- MSE for children – DSM Zero to Three, revised
  - Incorporates
    - Developmental assessment
    - Use of fantasy
    - Concept of self
    - Estimated IQ
    - Neuromuscular integration
    - Awareness of problem

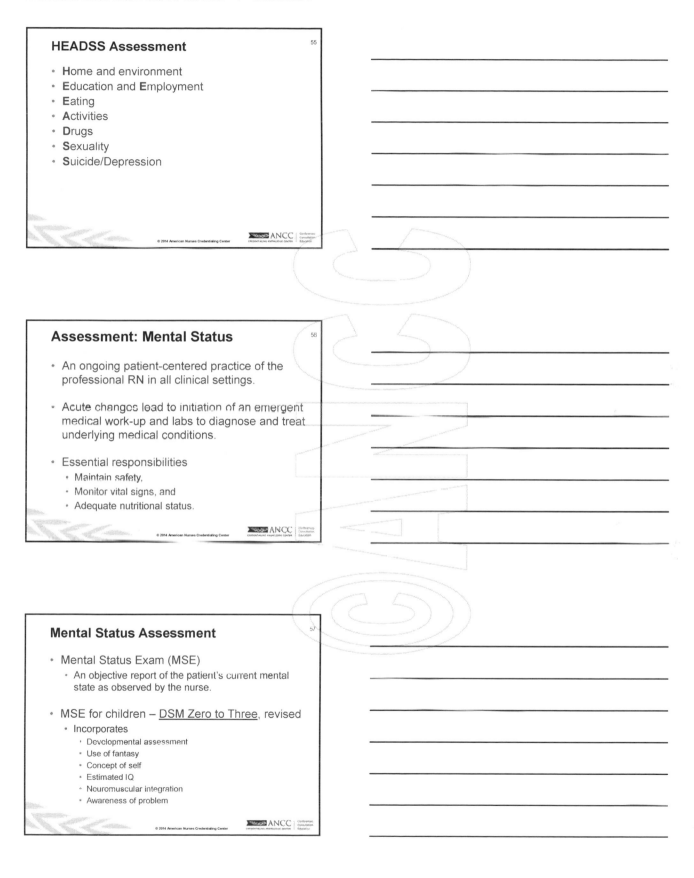

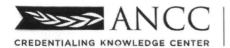
Seven MSE Components 58

1. General appearance and behavior
2. Mood and affect (emotional state)
3. Thought content and thought process
4. Senses and perceptions
5. Sensorium: Level of consciousness
6. Cognition and memory
7. Judgment and insight

© 2014 American Nurses Credentialing Center

MSE: Appearance and Behavior 59

- Overall appearance related to age and culture
- Hygiene and grooming
- Appropriateness of clothing to age, style, weather, and occasion (setting or location)
- Posture and mannerisms (eye contact?)
- General behavior (impulsivity, passive, hostile, fearful)
- Motor behavior (pacing, lethargic, catatonic, echopraxia, tics)
- Attitude toward nurse willingness to cooperate

© 2014 American Nurses Credentialing Center

MSE: Mood and Affect 60

- Mood: statement of internal feelings that influence behavior (e.g., "I feel depressed," "I feel good").

- Affect: observation of emotional expression and variations noted in facial, vocal, body language (e.g., flat, guarded, inappropriate, blunted, restricted, labile, looks suspicious, appears elated).

- Are mood and affect congruent or incongruent?

© 2014 American Nurses Credentialing Center

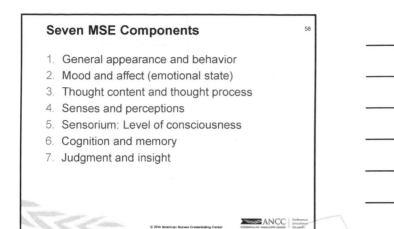

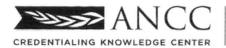

MSE: Thought Content

61

- Patient has to "talk" in order for nurse to assess content in order to find out what's on patient's mind or what patient thinking.
- Suicide: Plan, opportunity, means?
- Homicide: Victim, realistic plan?
- Delusions: Fixed, false beliefs?
- Phobias: Intense and unreasonable fear?
- Obsessions: Intrusive, repetitious, or patterned?
- Insight: Realization of problem, the "Ah-ha!" moment.
- Judgment: Decision-making or foresight

© 2014 American Nurses Credentialing Center

MSE: Thought Content

62

- Delusions: False, fixed beliefs that are incongruent with normative culture or religious beliefs.
  - Of reference: Believe others thoughts, words or actions refer to self (patient).
  - Persecution: Believe others have malevolent intentions toward self (patient), or are conspiring against the person (patient).
  - Religious: Unrealistic special relationship with God.
  - Nihilistic: Destruction of self, world, or body part, belief one is dead.
  - Grandiose: Believes is special, gifted, powerful, or important without factual support.

© 2014 American Nurses Credentialing Center

MSE: Thought Processes

63

- Does patient seem to understand what is said? Does patient respond appropriately, or is it delayed or rapidly/impulsively delivered?
- Continuity and organization of ideas
  - Problems with word finding or unexpected thought blockage?
  - Problems with processing abstract ideas?
  - Flow and rhythm: Slowed or racing thoughts?
  - Ideas are coherent, logical, illogical?
  - Amount: Excessive or poverty of speech?
  - Language used or special meanings?

© 2014 American Nurses Credentialing Center

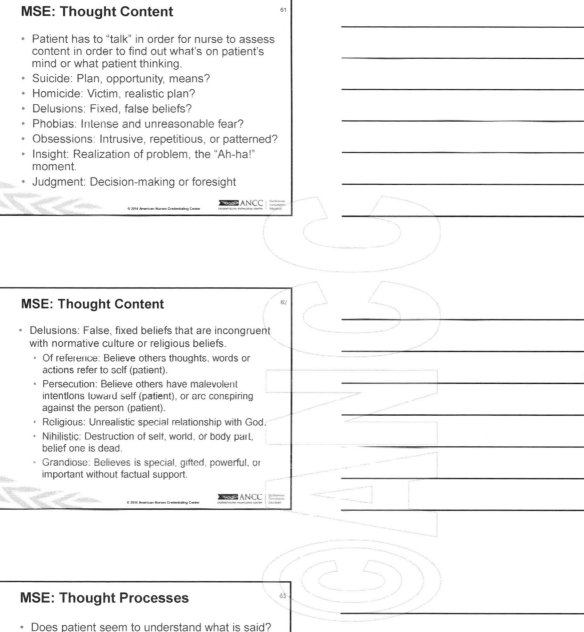

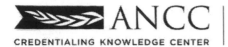
MSE: Thought Processing Language Deficits [64]

- Clanging
  - Words chosen based on similar sounds (rhyming), not associated ideas.
- Echolalia
  - Repetition of words or phrases heard from others.
- Neologisms
  - Creation of new words that don't make sense.
- Word Salad
  - Disorganized, mixed-up, or senseless progression of words.
- Perseveration
  - Tedious repetition of the same words or ideas regardless of stimuli.

© 2014 American Nurses Credentialing Center

MSE: Thought Processing Language Deficits [65]

- Flight of ideas
  - Ideas not logically connected, abrupt changes in topic.
- Loose associations
  - Limited or no logical connection between words or ideas.
- Circumstantial
  - Excessive and unnecessary detail, may eventually answer the question.
- Tangential
  - Never returns to the point or answer the question.
- Thought blocking
  - Interruption or delay in thought processing, not related to lack of concentration, distraction, or anxiety.

© 2014 American Nurses Credentialing Center

MSE: Perceptual Alterations [66]

- Depersonalization
  - Feeling detached as if one is an outside observer of one's mental processes or body.
- Hallucinations
  - Sensory-perceptual alteration in one or more of the five senses.
- Illusions
  - False perception a misinterpretation of a stimuli.
- Déjà vu or flashbacks
  - Sense of being there before or knowing someone from before.

© 2014 American Nurses Credentialing Center

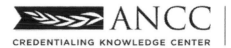
MSE: Connecting Sensory-Perceptual Alterations with Possible Etiologies

67

- Schizophrenia
  - Auditory, visual, or somatic hallucinations
  - Mood incongruence
  - Bizarre command
- Depression/Mania
  - Mood congruence with thoughts
- Dementia
  - Visual hallucinations
- Acute alcohol withdrawal
  - Tactile hallucinations
- Seizures
  - Olfactory hallucinations
  - Gustatory hallucinations

© 2014 American Nurses Credentialing Center

MSE: Sensorium, Cognition, Memory

68

- Sensorium
  - Level of consciousness

- Cognition
  - Orientation to person, time, and place
  - Abstract thinking ability
  - Concentration ability: Serial 7s (keep in mind educational level)

- Memory recall
  - Immediate
  - Recent
  - Remote

© 2014 American Nurses Credentialing Center

MSE: Judgment and Insight

69

- Judgment
  - Realistic decision-making based on:
    - Current level of knowledge
    - Realistic understanding of options
    - Resources and educational level
    - Strengths and limitations.

- Insight
  - Extent of one's awareness of own problem.
  - Willingness to look at one's role in maintaining symptoms.
  - Awareness of:
    - Behavioral consequences
    - Lifestyle changes needed for enhanced coping.

© 2014 American Nurses Credentialing Center

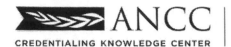

Mini-Mental Status Examination (MMSE)   70

- 30-item "point-in-time" tool to assess cognition.
  - Easily administered (takes 5 to 10 mins.)
  - Rapid fluctuations can be observed
  - Score ranges from 0 to 30 with lower scores indicating greater impairment
    - Score 18 to 23 suggests mild to moderate cognitive impairment
    - Score 15 to 17 or less suggests severe impairment
- Mental status impairments are suggestive of possible organic dysfunction. Many potential etiologies that have to be ruled out (medications, use of substances, fluid/electrolyte imbalances, and cognitive disorder).
- A major cause of medical morbidity and mortality!

© 2014 American Nurses Credentialing Center

Physical Examination Assessment Skills   71

- Auscultation
  - Listen to sounds produced by the body.
- Inspection
  - Direct observation of body areas.
- Palpation
  - Light touch with gentle pressure can detect areas of irregularity and tenderness.
  - Deep touch can assess the condition of underlying organs.
- Percussion
  - Tapping the body with fingertips to evaluate size, borders, and consistency of body organs.

© 2014 American Nurses Credentialing Center

Assessment Review of Systems   72

- Document the presence or absence of findings related to each major body system: "How is your/your child's…?"
  - Neurological: Cranial nerves, reflexes, and sensorium
  - Endocrine: Breasts, menarche, and hormonal functions
  - Hematologic: Hematology, immunology
  - Respiratory: Thorax and lungs, head and neck
  - Cardiovascular: Rates, rhythms, vasculature, and distention
  - Gastrointestinal: Height, weight, BMI, appetite/nutrition, elimination, and abdomen
  - Integumentary: Temperature, flushing, tone, rash, skin, hair, nails, and evidence of lesions/bruises
  - Genitourinary: Genitalia, reproductive organs, Tanner stage
  - Musculoskeletal: Muscular tone, strength, movement, fractures, curvatures, assistive devices, and pain

© 2014 American Nurses Credentialing Center

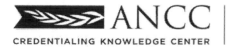
Cranial Nerves Assessment

73

• On	I.	Olfactory—smell
• Old	II.	Optic—central vision
• Olympus	III.	Oculomotor—eye movement, corneal reflex
Towering	IV.	Trochlear—eye movement
• Top	V.	Trigeminal—chews systematically
• A	VI.	Abducens—eye movement
• Fen	VII.	Facial—facial movement
• And	VIII.	Acoustic—hearing
• German	IX.	Glossopharyngeal
• Viewed	X.	Vagus—can make guttural sound
• Some	XI.	Spinal Accessory—shrug shoulders
• Hops	XII.	Hypoglossal—stick out tongue

© 2014 American Nurses Credentialing Center

Neurological Assessment

74

Glasgow Coma Scale		
Eyes Open	Spontaneously	4
	To verbal command	3
	To pain	2
	No response	1
Command/Pain	Obeys	6
	Localizes pain	5
	Flexion: Withdrawal	4
	Flexion: Abnormal (decorticate rigidity)	3
	Extension (decerebrate rigidity)	2
	No response	1
Verbal Response	Oriented and converses	5
	Disoriented and converses	4
	Inappropriate words	3
	Incomprehensible sounds	2
	No response	1
	TOTAL	

Reflexes

* Biceps, triceps, brachioradialis, patellar, Achilles, and plantar; Babinski reflex is normal in infants
* Pupils (reactive or non-reactive)
* Grip strength

© 2014 American Nurses Credentialing Center

Assessment: Vital Signs

75

* Critical data the professional RN considers in daily nursing care and treatment planning.

Temperature
* Oral: 37° C/98.6° F

Pulse rate
* Infant 120 to 160 bpm
* Child: 75 to 100 bpm
* Adolescent: 60 to 90 bpm
* Adult: 60 to 100 bpm

Blood pressure
* 1 yr.: 95/65; 10 yr. 110/65
* Adolescent: 120/75
* Adult: 120/80, Elder:140/90
* Hypertension (Adult): 140/90 or above

Respiratory rate
* Six months: 30 to 50
* 2 yrs.: 25 to 32
* Child: 20 to 30
* Adolescent: 16 to 19
* Adult: 12 to 20

© 2014 American Nurses Credentialing Center

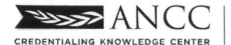

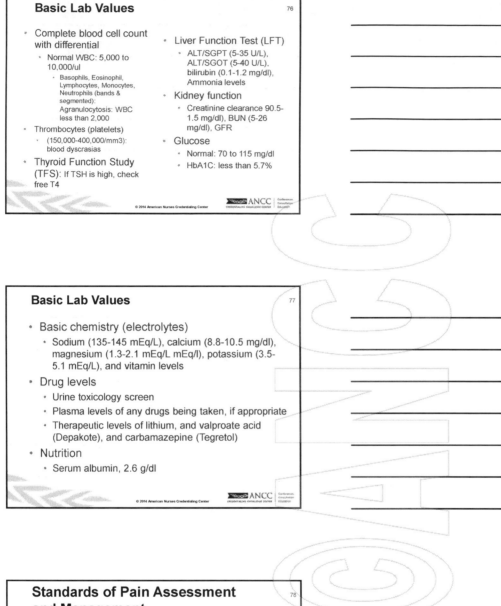

Basic Lab Values 76

- Complete blood cell count with differential
  - Normal WBC: 5,000 to 10,000/ul
    - Basophils, Eosinophil, Lymphocytes, Monocytes, Neutrophils (bands & segmented): Agranulocytosis: WBC less than 2,000
- Thrombocytes (platelets)
  - (150,000-400,000/mm3): blood dyscrasias
- Thyroid Function Study (TFS): If TSH is high, check free T4
- Liver Function Test (LFT)
  - ALT/SGPT (5-35 U/L), ALT/SGOT (5-40 U/L), bilirubin (0.1-1.2 mg/dl), Ammonia levels
- Kidney function
  - Creatinine clearance 90.5-1.5 mg/dl), BUN (5-26 mg/dl), GFR
- Glucose
  - Normal: 70 to 115 mg/dl
  - HbA1C: less than 5.7%

© 2014 American Nurses Credentialing Center

Basic Lab Values 77

- Basic chemistry (electrolytes)
  - Sodium (135-145 mEq/L), calcium (8.8-10.5 mg/dl), magnesium (1.3-2.1 mEq/L mEq/l), potassium (3.5-5.1 mEq/L), and vitamin levels
- Drug levels
  - Urine toxicology screen
  - Plasma levels of any drugs being taken, if appropriate
  - Therapeutic levels of lithium, and valproate acid (Depakote), and carbamazepine (Tegretol)
- Nutrition
  - Serum albumin, 2.6 g/dl

© 2014 American Nurses Credentialing Center

Standards of Pain Assessment and Management 78

- Patient has a right to be pain free
- A Critical Role for the Registered Nurse
  - Assess pain existence, nature, and intensity
    - History: Onset, location, intensity, and medical history
  - Observe pain characteristics
    - Vocalizations
    - Facial expressions
    - Body movement
    - Desire for social interaction
  - Determine patient's perception of pain
    - Meaning: Potential factors that may affect pain experience (loneliness, potentially fatal medical illness)
  - Effects on physical, sexual, emotional/psychological, and social functioning (secondary gain?)

© 2014 American Nurses Credentialing Center

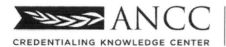

Standards of Pain Assessment and Management

79

- Record pain assessment results so regular reassessment and follow-up is facilitated.
- Determine and assure staff competency in pain assessment and management.
- Establish policies/procedures that support appropriate prescriptions, timely receipt, and administration of effective pain medications.
- Educate patients about effective pain management (prescriptions, complementary/integrative therapies).
- Address patient needs for symptom management in discharge planning.
- Maintain a pain control performance improvement plan.

© 2014 American Nurses Credentialing Center

Nutritional Assessment

80

- USDA: Evidence-based advice promotes health and reduces risk for major chronic diseases through diet and physical activity.
  - www.chosemyplate.gov
- No lab tests that effectively measure nutritional status.
- Body weight 15% or more below expected weight for age and height should receive further work-up to differentiate eating disorder vs. medical disorder.
- Recent weight loss
  - Depression (with loss of appetite), Hyperthyroidism?
- Recent weight gain
  - Taking antidepressants, anticonvulsants, Lithium, or antipsychotics?

© 2014 American Nurses Credentialing Center

Nutritional Assessment

81

- Tools
  - Body Mass Index (BMI): calculation ratio from height/weight
    http://www.cdc.gov/nccdphp/dnpa/bmi/index.htm
    - Normal: BMI 20 to 25
    - Overweight: BMI 25 to 29
    - Obese: BMI 30 to 35
  - Ideal body weight growth charts or formulas for infants and children
  - 24-hour food history or 3-7 day food diaries
  - Food/fluid intake measures
  - Physical assessment, skin turgor
  - Lab values: Serum albumin, others
  - Knowledge of nutrition and personal preferences
  - Supplements, prescriptions, alcohol, and drugs

© 2014 American Nurses Credentialing Center

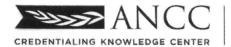 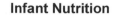
Infant Nutrition

82

- American Academy of Pediatrics recommends breast feeding for first year of life.
  - Caution if mother is on psychotropic medications or HIV positive.

- Birth weight doubles at 4 to 5 months and triples by one year (developmental milestones).

- Calorie needs:
  - Higher in 1st 6 months - 108 kcal/kg of body weight
  - Less in 2nd 6 months - 98 kcal/kg

© 2014 American Nurses Credentialing Center

USDA* Guidelines: Ages 2 and older

83

- Provide adequate nutrients within calorie needs
  - Need to consume a variety of nutrient-dense foods and beverages.
- Weight management
  - To prevent gradual weight gain over time, make small decreases in food and beverage calories and increase physical activity.
- Physical activity
  - To reduce risk of chronic disease in adulthood, engage in at least 30 minutes of moderate intensity physical activity on most days; 60 minutes or more for children or adults who need to manage weight

- *USDA=U.S. Department of Agriculture

© 2014 American Nurses Credentialing Center

Sleep: Opportunity for Parasympathetic Restoration

84

- Sleep quality and amount is important.
- Sleep needs change over the lifespan.
  - Children under 10 years of age need 10 hours or more.
  - Children over 10 years of age need 9 hours or more.
  - Adults needs vary; daytime functioning is key.
- Sleep difficulties: 20 to 30% of adults report having sleep difficulties
- Sleep disorders
  - Insomnia, hypersomnia, (many other sleep disorders recognized by the National Sleep Foundation
- Insomnia: the complaint of sleep that is insufficient to support good daytime functioning.

© 2014 American Nurses Credentialing Center

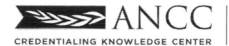
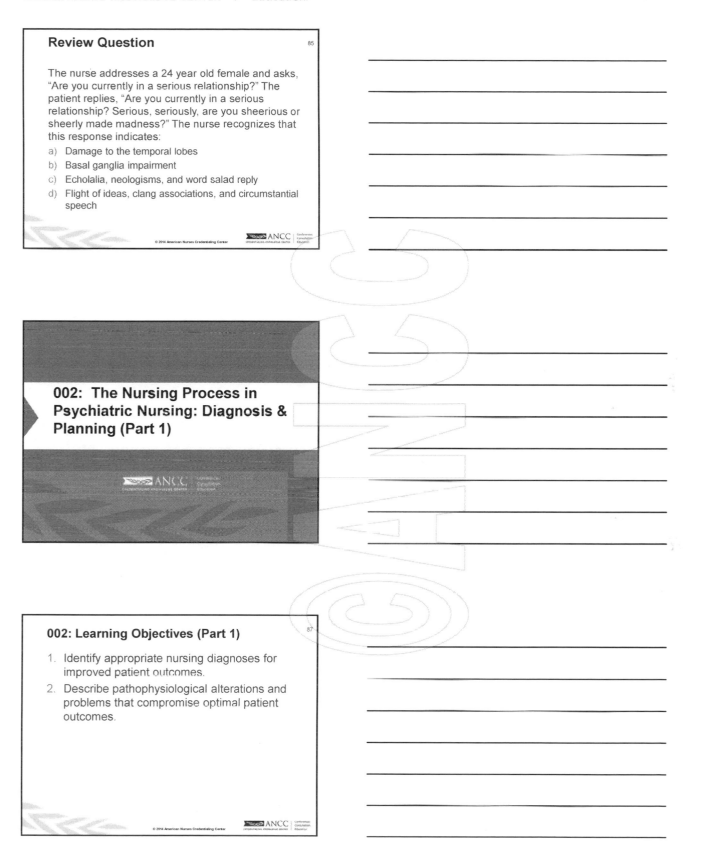

Review Question
85

The nurse addresses a 24 year old female and asks, "Are you currently in a serious relationship?" The patient replies, "Are you currently in a serious relationship? Serious, seriously, are you sheerious or sheerly made madness?" The nurse recognizes that this response indicates:

a) Damage to the temporal lobes
b) Basal ganglia impairment
c) Echolalia, neologisms, and word salad reply
d) Flight of ideas, clang associations, and circumstantial speech

© 2014 American Nurses Credentialing Center

002: The Nursing Process in Psychiatric Nursing: Diagnosis & Planning (Part 1)

002: Learning Objectives (Part 1)
87

1. Identify appropriate nursing diagnoses for improved patient outcomes.
2. Describe pathophysiological alterations and problems that compromise optimal patient outcomes.

© 2014 American Nurses Credentialing Center

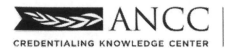
General Survey Across the Lifespan 88

- **Infant:** Parent-infant interactions/touch, feeding, and cry
- **Early childhood:** Mood, nutritional state, speech, cry, facial expression, developmental and chronologic age, skills, parent-child interactions, separation, tolerance, affection, and discipline
- **Late childhood:** Orientation to time and place; factual knowledge; language and number skills: motor skills used for writing, tying laces, buttoning, and drawing
- **Adult:** Observe general state of health, height, build, sexual development (Tanner stage), posture, motor activity, gait, dress, grooming, personal hygiene, odors, affect, reactions, speech, level of consciousness, and mental status

© 2014 American Nurses Credentialing Center

Sexual Health Across the Lifespan 89

- Infants: Initial body exploration
- Toddler/Preschooler: Gender identity development
- School-aged: Same sex peer groups, increased need for privacy
- Adolescence: Onset of secondary sex signs and exploration of sexual orientation, body image issues
    - Girls: Average age for menarche (menses) is 12
    - Boys: Ejaculation between 12 and 14; nocturnal emissions
- Adulthood: Continue to develop intimacy and sexuality
- Middle aged: Menopause (ages 48 and 52); andropause
- Elders: Declining health and hormonal changes, healthy sexuality/sex still possible

© 2014 American Nurses Credentialing Center

Physical/Emotional Changes: Puberty 90

- Sexual History Assessment
    - "Are you sexually active?"
    - "Do you have sex with men, women, or both?" www.cdc.gov/std/treatment/SexualHistory.pdf
    - "Do you practice safe sex every time?"
    - "Are you in a monogamous relationship?"
    - Growth in gonads, secondary sex characteristics
- Emotional tasks of adolescents include:
    - Achieving body mastery, controlling sexual and aggressive urges, separating from family, achieving sense of identity.
- Physical height spurt apparent:
    - Girls: 10 to 14 years
    - Boys: 10.5 to 17.5 years

© 2014 American Nurses Credentialing Center

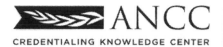
Physical Changes: Aging Process   91

- CNS
  - Decrease in neurons and some neurotransmitters, however, continued ability to form new synapses.
  - Brain becomes smaller and lighter.
  - Varying degree of vision and hearing loss.
- Cardiovascular
  - Heart and blood vessels stiffen (sclerosis).
  - Cardiac output declines.
  - Hemodynamic instabilities (hypo-/hypertension).
- Respiratory
  - Decline in respiratory muscle strength and control of breathing.

© 2014 American Nurses Credentialing Center

Physical Changes: Aging Process   92

- Gastrointestinal
  - Decreased hepatic blood flow may decrease drug clearance.
  - Presence of Geriatric Failure to Thrive (GFF): Polypharmacy.
- Endocrine
  - Changes in production of most hormones, change in function may not occur.
- Musculoskeletal
  - Decline in muscle mass with increasing weakness.
  - Presence of bone loss (osteoporosis or osteopenia).

© 2014 American Nurses Credentialing Center

Physical Changes: Aging Process   93

- Hematological and Immune
  - Decreased ability of bone marrow to produce red blood cells with blood loss.
- Renal
  - Decreased size
  - Decreased renal blood flow
  - Decreased function
    - Creatinine clearance declines, Blood urea nitrogen (BUN) Glomerular Filtration Rate (GFR)

© 2014 American Nurses Credentialing Center

Assessment: Psychosis

94

- Scale:
  - Positive and Negative Syndrome Scale (PANSS)

- Evidence of perceptual alterations, disturbed thoughts, contents, and processes

_____

_____

_____

_____

_____

_____

Assessment: Mood Symptom Severity

95

- Anxiety scales
  - Hamilton Anxiety Scale
  - Multidimensional Anxiety Scale for Children (MASC)

- Depression scales
  - Hamilton Depression Scale
  - Beck Depression Inventory (BDI), Adult and Child versions
  - Children's Depression Rating Scale (CDRS)
  - Geriatric Depression Scale

- These are some examples. There are many more.

_____

_____

_____

_____

Assessment: Suicidal Ideation (SI)

96

- Components of a Lethality Assessment
  - Past history, previous attempt: At higher risk if positive
  - Plan and means: Are weapons available?
  - Unwillingness of patient to contract for safety.
- Determine level of risk based on presence of individual or co-occurring factors
  - Hopelessness, depression, substance user, impulsive personality, self-hatred, thought disorder, elder white widowed male, adolescent, and history of abuse or neglect.

_____

_____

_____

_____

_____

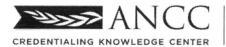
Assessment: Suicidal Ideation (SI) cont. 97

- Identify family or social/environmental factors/supports
  - Difficult home situation, parental rejection or indifference, poor social support, isolation, few social, vocational, or educational opportunities, and firearms/weapons in the home.

© 2014 American Nurses Credentialing Center

Assessment: Abuse and Neglect 98

Behavioral evidence:

- Difficulty managing school, work, or parenting responsibilities
- Anxiety, depression, extreme mood changes, or withdrawal
- Low self-esteem or poor self-image
- Decreased attention span
- Self-mutilation
- Promiscuity
- Parental indifference
- Enuresis or encopresis

Physical evidence:

- Bruising on padded body areas or rawness, itching in perianal area or inner thigh
- Unexplained injuries or a history/presence of multiple fractures
- Burns or bite marks
- Neglect, evidenced by poor care
- Presence of a sexually transmitted infection
- Unusual incidence of urinary tract infections

Sexual Assault Nurse Examiner (SANE) and medical forensics team may need to be involved.

© 2014 American Nurses Credentialing Center

CATEGORY I B: PROBLEM IDENTIFICATION AND NURSING DIAGNOSIS

© 2014 American Nurses Credentialing Center

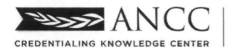
Nursing Diagnoses: Practice Standard 2

100

- Professional RN analyzes and synthesizes assessment data to formulate patient-specific nursing diagnoses from identified problems.
  - Allows recognition of emergent and urgent problems, patterns, and trends in comparison with normal standards.
  - Provides for prioritization and direction of treatment.

- North American Nursing Diagnosis Association – International (NANDA-I) classification system
  - Statements of problem(s) treatable by nursing interventions (published 2012-2014).

© 2014 American Nurses Credentialing Center · ANCC

Nursing Diagnoses: Practice Standard 2

101

- NANDA-I examples
  - Risk for suicide
  - Risk for self-mutilation
  - Inefficient denial
  - Risk for violence or injury
  - Noncompliance with medication or treatment
  - Fear
  - Hopelessness
  - Sleep pattern disturbance

- NANDA-I examples
  - Dysfunctional grieving
  - Rape-trauma syndrome
  - Self-care deficit
  - Spiritual distress
  - Altered urinary elimination
  - Ineffective individual coping
  - Ineffective family coping

Avoid prejudicial, judgmental, stigmatizing statements.

Highest priorities are listed first.

© 2014 American Nurses Credentialing Center · ANCC

Critical Thinking: Prioritizing Nursing Care Using Maslow

102

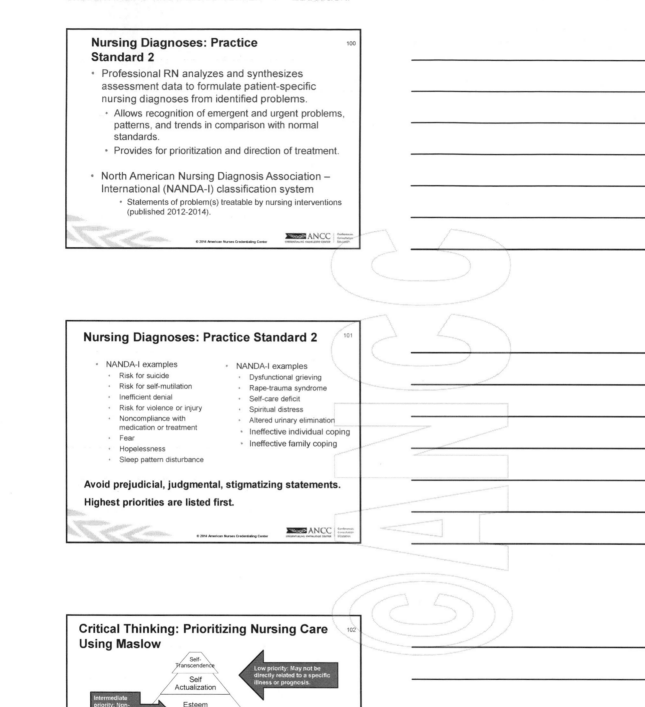

Maslow's Hierarchy of Needs and Nursing Priorities

I can feel guilty about the past, apprehensive about the future, but only in the present can I act. The ability to be in the present moment is a major component of mental wellness.
Abraham Maslow

© 2014 American Nurses Credentialing Center · ANCC

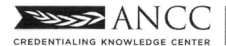
Critical Assessment Priority Areas

103

- Problem-based or behavioral-based priorities:
  - Suicide (self-directed violence)/Homicide (other-directed violence)
  - Aggression
  - Partner/Domestic abuse
  - Falls
  - Pain

- Symptom-based priorities:
  - Acute mental changes (e.g., confusion, rapid speech)
  - Somatic (e.g., cardiac, respiratory, movement)

© 2014 American Nurses Credentialing Center

Suicide and Self-Harm Risk

104

- Suicide: 3rd leading cause of death in adolescents between ages 10 and 24; 10th leading cause among ages 10+ (CDC 2009).
- Greatest increase during 1999-2010 among Asian/Pacific Islanders, followed by Whites (CDC).
- Warning signs (persist for 1 month or more).
  - Loss of initiative
  - Alcohol/drug use
  - Loneliness; feeling alone, sadness, crying; withdrawal from family and friends; decrease in school performance
  - History of impulsive behavior
  - Firearms available
  - Appetite, sleep disturbances
  - Verbalization of suicidal thoughts
- Self-Mutilation (DSM-5: Nonsuicidal Self-Injury [NSSI]).

© 2014 American Nurses Credentialing Center

Problem: Suicidal and Self-Harm Risk

105

- Lethality Assessment: A critical role for the professional RN
  - High Risk (1:1 status): Patient has highly lethal plan with actual or potential access; is a high elopement risk; has constant SI with history of past attempts. Patient is unwilling to contract for safety and voices hopelessness.

  - Moderate Risk (q15 min. status): Patient ambivalent; has plan, but no access; is a low elopement risk, may have intermittent SI; and with past attempts of low lethality.

  - Low Risk (no precautions): No plan; 0 to 2 symptoms, rare SI

    - Stuart & Laria, 2005

© 2014 American Nurses Credentialing Center

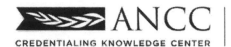

Problem: Homicidal Ideation (HI)

106

- Homicide is 2nd leading cause of death among 15-24 year olds (CDC, 2010).
- CDC (2010): Homicide is leading cause among 10-24 year old black males, the 2nd cause for American Indians/Alaskan Natives, and 3rd for Hispanics.
- Violence:
  - Is a negative function or destructive use of anger,
  - Threatens or injures other's security,
  - Includes injuries that can be physical or verbal, and
  - Is designed to punish, cause pain, or ignore other's rights.

© 2014 American Nurses Credentialing Center

Problem: Abuse, Assault, and Aggression

107

- Purpose: Intent to dominate, manipulate, intimidate or control a more vulnerable person; exhibit power and/or control. These acts are often hidden from society.
- Types:
  - Physical or Sexual: Beating, starving, torturing, non-consensual rape, or incest.
  - Emotional or Verbal: Spoken words or behaviors that belittle, acts of stalking, attacks on self-esteem, attempts to humiliate, scapegoat or intimidate. Usually conducted against a vulnerable person (child, elder, dependent partner, homeless person).

© 2014 American Nurses Credentialing Center

Problem: Partner/Domestic Violence

108

- Leading cause of injury to women ages 15 to 44 (reproductive age)
- Cycle of Assault
  - Triggering phase: Stress response occurs due to stress-producing event.
  - Escalation phase: Responses escalate behaviors leading to loss of control.
  - Crisis phase: Loss of control occurs both physically and emotionally.
  - Recovery phase: A cooling down time when the abuser slows down and returns to more normal responses.
  - Post-crisis depression phase: Abuser attempts reconciliation with others (Smith: 1981 in Keltner, et al. 2003).

© 2014 American Nurses Credentialing Center

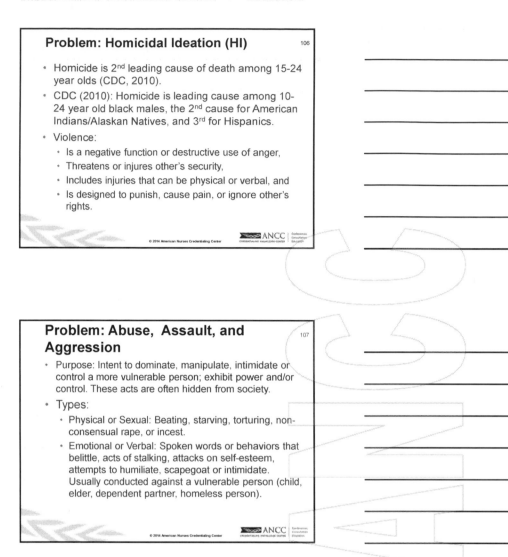

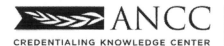
Problem: Aggression

109

- Observe for prodromal signs: Verbal/physical threats or actions directed toward property, animals, self, or others.
  - Biological theories: Brain damage (frontal lobe; traumatic brain injuries), intellectual or learning disabilities that impair ability to cope with frustration, delayed gratification, use of alcohol, or other disinhibiting substances.
  - Psychological theories: Severe emotional deprivation or overt rejection in childhood or parental seduction, exposure to violence in formative years, poor coping resources.
  - Sociocultural theories: Lack of interpersonal ties, poor bonding/attachment, learned behaviors.

© 2014 American Nurses Credentialing Center

Problem: Aggression

110

- Behavioral history
  - Childhood cruelty to animals or children.
  - Fire setting or similar dangerous actions.
  - Recent violent behavior toward self or others.
  - Recent accidents, threats, or poor judgment in potentially dangerous situations.
- Observable behavior and emotional responses
  - Escalating irritability, sensitivity, or hostility.
  - Altered states of consciousness/substance abuse.
  - Emotions: Severe rage/anger, or fear/panic.
  - Active psychotic symptoms with paranoid ideation.

© 2014 American Nurses Credentialing Center

NANDA-I: Suicide, Homicide, Abuse, Assault, and Aggression

111

- Risk for suicide/homicide
- Hopelessness
- Ineffective coping related to negative role modeling
- Risk for violence to others related to childhood environment of violence

© 2014 American Nurses Credentialing Center

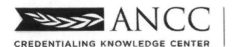
NANDA-I: Partner/Domestic Violence 112

- Ineffective (maladaptive) family coping, domestic violence/intimate abuse, and violence.
  - Vulnerable populations may include children, pregnant women, frail elders, and those with mental illness, cognitive impairments, developmental delays.
  - More pregnant women die as victims of domestic violence than from any other cause.
  - Perpetrators come from all walks of life and are likely to have grown up in violent home or exposed in community. Tend to have poor impulse control, low self-esteem, and dependent personalities.
  - View victims as their property.

Problem: Vital Signs Alterations 113

- Advanced age can lead to:
  - Increased sensitivity to environmental temperature
  - Increased risk for hypothermia
  - Increased BP tendencies, especially systolic due to decreased vessel elasticity
  - Decreased efficiency of respiratory muscles with increased breathlessness.
- Medication side effects can lead to:
  - Orthostatic hypotension.
    - Systolic falls to 90mmHg or below.
    - Measure BP supine, sitting, and standing prior to initiating medications.

Problem: Falls and Risk Conditions 114

- General: Over age 60, history of falls, history of smoking, alcohol, or drug abuse.
- Mental status: Lethargy, confusion, disorientation, inability to understand directions, impaired memory, or judgment.
- Physical conditions: Vertigo, unsteady gait, weight-bearing joint problems, weakness, paresis/paralysis, seizure disorder, impaired vision, impaired hearing, slow reaction times, diarrhea, urinary frequency, urgency, nocturia.

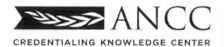
Problem: Falls and Risk Conditions cont. [115]

- Medications: Diuretics, psychotropics, hypotensive, or CNS depressants and medications that increase GI motility (e.g., laxatives).
- Ambulatory or other devices used: cane, crutches, walker, wheelchair, Geri chair, braces.

NANDA-I: Falls [116]

- Risk for self-harm related to postural imbalance.
- Impaired physical mobility.

Problem: Pain - The "Fifth" Vital Sign [117]

- Pain assessment: A critical role for the professional RN.

- TJC outlines Standards of Pain Management and recommends regular assessment and management.

- ABCDE

  - Ask about pain regularly. Assess pain systematically.

  - Believe patient and family in reports of pain and what relieves it.

  - Choose appropriate pain control options for patient, family, setting.

  - Deliver interventions in a timely, logical, and coordinated fashion.

  - Empower patients and families. Enable them to exercise some control to the greatest extent possible.

NANDA-I: Pain

118

- Anxiety
- Hopelessness
- Depressed mood
- Fear
- Mobility and impaired physical
- Pain: Acute and chronic
- Self-care deficit
- Sexual dysfunction
- Sleep pattern disturbance
- Caregiver role strain

© 2014 American Nurses Credentialing Center

Problem: Abnormal PE Findings Related to Psychiatric Disorders and Medications

119

- HEENT (head, eyes, ears, nose, throat)
  - Head
    - Progressively severe headache: R/0 hypertensive crisis due to tyramine interaction with MAOIs
  - Eyes (and vision):
    - Nystagmus: Substance intoxication, brain lesions
    - Oculogyric crisis: Neuroleptic induced dystonia
  - Ears (and hearing)
    - Diminished hearing: Normal aging, cauliflower ears
  - Throat
    - High fever and sore throat (assess WBC levels for Agranulocytosis)
    - Note masses, swollen glands, deviation of trachea, and thyroid enlargement (goiter)

© 2014 American Nurses Credentialing Center

Problem: Abnormal PE Findings Related to Psychiatric Disorders and Medications

120

- Neurological system
  - Tremors from lithium, anticonvulsants, or Parkinson's
  - Gait and balance disturbances: Encephalopathy
  - Neuroleptic Malignant Syndrome (NMS)
  - Change in mental status, delirium, weakness, numbness, or abnormal sensations
  - Extrapyramidal symptoms (EPS)
- Cardiovascular system
  - ECG changes (QT interval lengthening) from TCAs, neuroleptics
  - Orthostatic hypotension: TCAs, neuroleptics, or antihypertensives
  - Tachycardia from stimulants, anxiety, or anorexia
  - Hypertension from metabolic syndrome r/t antipsychotics
  - Bradycardia from beta-blockers, anorexia

© 2014 American Nurses Credentialing Center

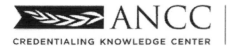
Problem: Abnormal PE Findings Related 121
to Psychiatric Disorders and Medications

* Respiratory system
  * Hyperventilation: Anxiety
* Endocrine system
  * Galactorrhea: Gynecomastia from neuroleptics/antipsychotics
  * Hypothyroidism: Depression
  * Diabetes: Neuroleptics/antipsychotics, obesity
  * Lactation: Antipsychotics
* Integumentary system
  * Stevens-Johnson Syndrome (toxic, potentially fatal epidermal necrolysis) from lamotrigine (Lamictal)

© 2014 American Nurses Credentialing Center

Problem: Abnormal PE Findings Related to 122
Psychiatric Disorders and Medications
(cont.)
* Gastrointestinal system
  * Hepatic cytochrome P450 (CYP 450) enzyme interactions can induce or inhibit the metabolism of certain drugs changing the desired concentration levels.
    * Nicotine is an inducer of liver enzymes.
* Genitourinary system
  * Renal disease or drugs that reduce renal clearance (e.g., NSAIDs) may increase serum concentration of drugs that are excreted by the kidneys (e.g., Lithium).
  * Question and document any signs of possible sexual abuse.

© 2014 American Nurses Credentialing Center

Problem: Abnormal PE Findings Related 123
to Psychiatric Disorders and Medications
(cont.)

* Musculoskeletal system
  * Body symmetry/Asymmetry: Dystonias, CVA, brain lesions
  * Abnormal movements: Extrapyramidal Symptoms (EPS)
    * Akathisia
    * Dyskinesias/Bradykinesia/Dystonia
    * Pseudoparkinsonism
    * Tardive dyskinesia
  * Gait disturbances
    * Ataxia: Alcoholic encephalopathy (Wernicke-Korsakoff's psychosis), substance use disorders, or dementia
    * Swallowing problems: Parkinson's Disease, dementia, or neuroleptic induced dystonia

© 2014 American Nurses Credentialing Center

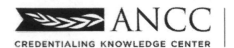
Problem: Abnormal PE Finding: Metabolic Syndrome

124

- Strongly associated with atypical neuroleptic (antipsychotic) medications
- Components of metabolic syndrome
  - Abdominal obesity
  - Atherogenic dyslipidemia
  - Elevated blood pressure
  - Insulin resistance with or without glucose intolerance
  - Proinflammatory state
  - Prothrombotic state
- Metabolic syndrome increases the risk for premature coronary heart disease.
  - Why Do Psychiatric Patients Die Sooner? (NASMPHD)

Problem: Sexually Transmitted Infections

125

- Syphilis
- Gonorrhea
- Chlamydia
- Trichomoniasis
- Human papillomavirus (HPV): Genital warts
- Herpes Simplex Virus (HSV): Vaccine available
- Human Immunodeficiency Virus (HIV): Rising among those age 50+

Problem: Human Immunodeficiency Virus

126

- Transmission routes: blood and other body fluids
  - Sexual contact, contaminated IV needles, transfusions
  - Universal Precautions mandated
- Pathophysiology
  - Virus targets the CD4 receptor on T4 lymphocytes.
  - Virus injects its RNA into the infected lymphocyte and becomes part of cell division, eventually disabling the patient's T4 lymphocytes.
- Vulnerable (higher risk) populations:
  - Gay men
  - IV drug users
  - Hemophiliacs
  - Unprotected sex behaviors
  - Children born to HIV+ women
  - Older adults

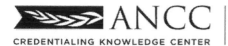
Problem: Acquired Immune Deficiency Syndrome

127

- About 6 months after initial HIV exposure, patients can test positive for HIV, those at risk need to be tested every 6 months.
- AIDS diagnosed
  - When CD4 ("helper cells") concentration falls to less than 200 cells/mm3.
  - Following an opportunistic infection, sometimes 10 to 17 yrs. after exposure.
  - Effective antiretroviral therapies have improved longevity and helps prevent opportunistic infections.

© 2014 American Nurses Credentialing Center

Problem: Gender Dysphoria

128

- Describes one's personal desire to be treated as a member of the opposite sex than what has been biologically assigned.
  - Manifests as personal convictions that one has typical feelings, thoughts, and behaviors of the other gender.
  - Desire to transform sex characteristics often accompanies these self-perceptions.
- Sexual orientation describes the sexual preference(s) of the person.

© 2014 American Nurses Credentialing Center

Review Question

129

What phrase or term describes the preferential desires of a person's sexual choice?

a) Sexual orientation
b) Bisexuality
c) Sexual dysfunction
d) Gender identity confusion

© 2014 American Nurses Credentialing Center

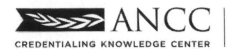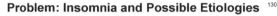

Problem: Insomnia and Possible Etiologies [130]

- Physical conditions
  - Parkinson's, cognitive disorders, sleep apnea, cardiovascular disorders, hyperthyroidism, diabetes, esophageal reflux, urinary frequency/infections, pain/discomfort, CNS stimulants, some antidepressants, anti-arrhythmic drugs, corticosteroids, thyroid medications, diuretics, rebound insomnia from overuse of sleeping pills, anxiety disorders, and stress.
- Altered sleep schedules
  - Hypervigilance, anxiety, mood/anxiety disorders, fear, psychoses.
- Environmental conditions
  - Travel, shift work, sundowner's syndrome, hospitalizations (noise/lights changes).

© 2014 American Nurses Credentialing Center

Review Question [131]

Which nursing diagnosis would specifically relate to a patient who states, "Don't waste that meal on me. I am already dead. I have no innards."

a) Risk for self-mutilation
b) Acute confusion
c) Disturbed thought content
d) Risk for disturbed human identity

© 2014 American Nurses Credentialing Center

Medical Conditions Affected by Psychological Factors [132]

Cardiovascular
- Migraine
- Essential hypertension
- Angina
- Tension headaches

Musculoskeletal
- Rheumatoid arthritis
- Low back pain

Respiratory
- Hyperventilation
- Asthma

Endocrine
- Hyperthyroidism
- Diabetes

Gastrointestinal
- Anorexia
- Peptic ulcer
- Irritable bowel syndrome
- Colitis
- Obesity

Integumentary
- Neurodermatitis
- Eczema
- Psoriasis
- Pruritus

Genitourinary
- Impotence
- Frigidity
- Premenstrual syndrome

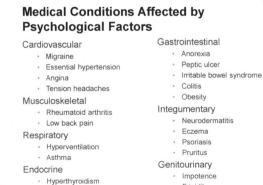

© 2014 American Nurses Credentialing Center

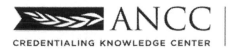
Medical Conditions Mimic Psychiatric Symptoms

133

- Hyperthyroidism: Nervous, irritable, insomnia, pressured speech, fear, impending death, anxiety disorders, and psychosis (heat intolerance, diaphoresis, tremor)
- Hypothyroidism: Lethargy, depressed, anxiety disorders, paranoia, and psychosis, (cold intolerance, dry skin, apathy)
- Hyperglycemia: Anxiety, agitation, delirium, and acetone breath
- Frontal Lobe Syndrome: Mood/personality changes and irritability
- Cushing's Syndrome: depression, insomnia, emotional lability, mania, and psychosis
- Adrenocorticotical insufficiency: Lethargy, depression, psychosis, delirium, anorexia, and nausea/vomiting

© 2014 American Nurses Credentialing Center

Medical Conditions Mimic Psychiatric Symptoms

134

- AIDS: Depression, personality changes, impaired memory, mutism, progressive dementia, mania, delirium
- Multiple Sclerosis: Anxiety, depression, euphoria, ataxia, muscle weakness, diffuse neuro signs with exacerbations and remissions
- Thiamine deficiency: Confusion, confabulation, decreased concentration, neuropathy, Wernicke-Korsakoff's psychosis
- Vitamin B12 deficiency: Irritability, pallor, dizziness, ataxia, fatigue
- Tumor: Judgment, seizures, loss of speech, or smell

© 2014 American Nurses Credentialing Center

135

UNDERSTANDING AND MANAGING EUSTRESS, DISTRESS, AND ANXIETY

© 2014 American Nurses Credentialing Center

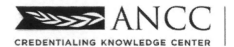
Eustress and Distress

136

- Stress is a normal life occurrence and is to be expected ("eu"=good; "dis"=bad).
- Hans Selye (1956) defined stress as a universal response.
- Stress responses are based on the meaning of the stressor, past experiences, amount of stress felt, and past coping skills.
  - Stress results when perceived demands outweigh perceived capacity to adapt.

© 2014 American Nurses Credentialing Center

Stage of Alarm: Selye's General Adaptation Syndrome

137

- Stressor perceived. Body reacts with flight-or-fight response and activation of the Hypothalamic-Pituitary-Adrenal (HPA) axis.
  - Hypothalamus secretes CRH.
  - CRH stimulates pituitary to release ACTH.
  - ACTH stimulates adrenal gland to release cortisol.
  - All senses become hyper-alerted.
  - Anxiety increases in proportion to the perceived threat.
  - Either problem solving or freezing results.
- When the stressor remains unresolved, the person moves to the second stage.

© 2014 American Nurses Credentialing Center

Stage of Resistance: Selye's General Adaptation Syndrome

138

- Defense mechanisms and coping strategies are employed.

- Anxiety continues to increase in proportion to the stress; the problem is either solved or the person moves on to the next stage.

- Homeostatic mechanisms are taxed as the person tries to maintain control.

© 2014 American Nurses Credentialing Center

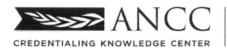

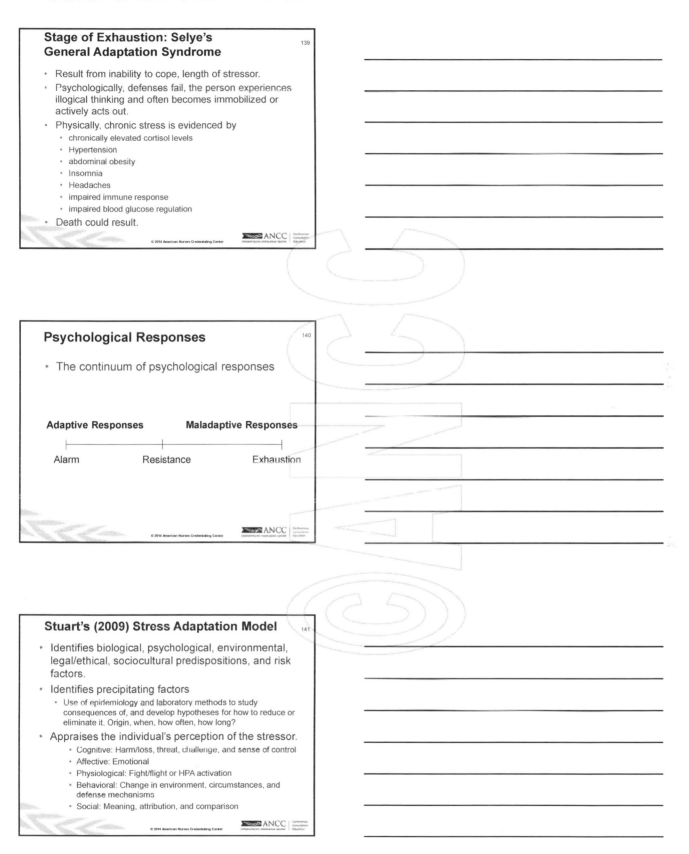

Stage of Exhaustion: Selye's General Adaptation Syndrome

139

- Result from inability to cope, length of stressor.
- Psychologically, defenses fail, the person experiences illogical thinking and often becomes immobilized or actively acts out.
- Physically, chronic stress is evidenced by
  - chronically elevated cortisol levels
  - Hypertension
  - abdominal obesity
  - Insomnia
  - Headaches
  - impaired immune response
  - impaired blood glucose regulation
- Death could result.

Psychological Responses

140

- The continuum of psychological responses

Adaptive Responses   **Maladaptive Responses**

| Alarm | Resistance | Exhaustion |

Stuart's (2009) Stress Adaptation Model

141

- Identifies biological, psychological, environmental, legal/ethical, sociocultural predispositions, and risk factors.
- Identifies precipitating factors
  - Use of epidemiology and laboratory methods to study consequences of, and develop hypotheses for how to reduce or eliminate it. Origin, when, how often, how long?
- Appraises the individual's perception of the stressor.
  - Cognitive: Harm/loss, threat, challenge, and sense of control
  - Affective: Emotional
  - Physiological: Fight/flight or HPA activation
  - Behavioral: Change in environment, circumstances, and defense mechanisms
  - Social: Meaning, attribution, and comparison

Stress Adaptation Model

142

- Factors that determine coping resources:
  - Personal abilities
  - Social support
  - Material assets
  - Positive beliefs

- Coping/defense mechanisms are efforts directed at stress management.
  - Problem-focused: Direct attempts to deal with the stressor
  - Cognitively focused: Attempts to change appraisal
  - Emotion-focused: Use of defense mechanisms

Stress Adaptation Model and Prevention

143

- Determine stage of treatment for implementation
  - Health promotion, Crisis, Acute, Maintenance
- Determine expected outcome
- Identify appropriate level of prevention effort.
  - Primary: Advocacy, psychoeducation, role modeling
  - Secondary: Screening
  - Tertiary: Optimal care

Stage of Treatment	Level of Prevention	Expected Outcome
Health Promotion	Primary	Optimal Well-being
Crisis	Secondary	Stabilization
Acute	Secondary	Remission
Maintenance	Tertiary	Recovery

Stress Management Techniques

144

- Cognitive
  - Cognitive restructuring
- Emotional
  - Journaling
  - Social support activities
  - Conflict resolution
- Behavioral
  - Learning what, and self-monitoring triggers or responses
  - Relaxation, breathing, mediation, prayer
  - Use of coping skills
- Physical
  - Diet and exercise
  - Sublimation through sports or other outlets

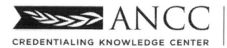
Psychophysiology and Pathophysiology   145

Psychophysiology: Branch of psychology concerned with the physiological bases of psychological processes.

Pathophysiology: Alterations in function that accompany a particular syndrome or disease.

- Psychotic (Thought) disorders
- Mood disorders
- Anxiety disorders
- Personality disorders
- Eating disorders
- Pervasive Developmental Disorders (PDD)
- Oppositional Defiance Disorder (ODD)

- Attention Deficit Hyperactivity Disorder (ADHD)
- Substance Use disorders
- Dementia
- Delirium
- Metabolic disorders
- Rett Syndrome
- Conduct Disorder (CD)

© 2014 American Nurses Credentialing Center

Two Hit Hypothesis of Psychiatric Disorders   146

- First Hit: Genetic vulnerability
  - Factors are inherited and create a risk for the development of psychiatric disorders.

- Second Hit: Environmental stressors
  - Stress triggers abnormal genes to produce abnormal gene products and illness.
  - Stressor can be due to physical (e.g., illness, viruses) or psychosocial (e.g., trauma, abuse, stress-related) causes.

  - Stahl. (2000). Essential psychopharmacology.

© 2011 American Nurses Credentialing Center

Heritability of Psychiatric Disorders   147

- Highest heritability
  - Schizophrenia (82 to 84%) (Kendler, 2001)
  - Bipolar disorder (85 to 89%) (McGuffin et al., 2003)

- Medium heritability
  - Alcoholism (52 to 58%) (Kendler, 2001)

- Lowest heritability
  - Anxiety disorders (37 to 43%) (Kendler, 2001)
  - Major depression (29 to 42%) (Kendler, Gatz, Gardner, Pedersen, 2006)

© 2014 American Nurses Credentialing Center

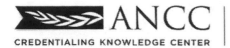
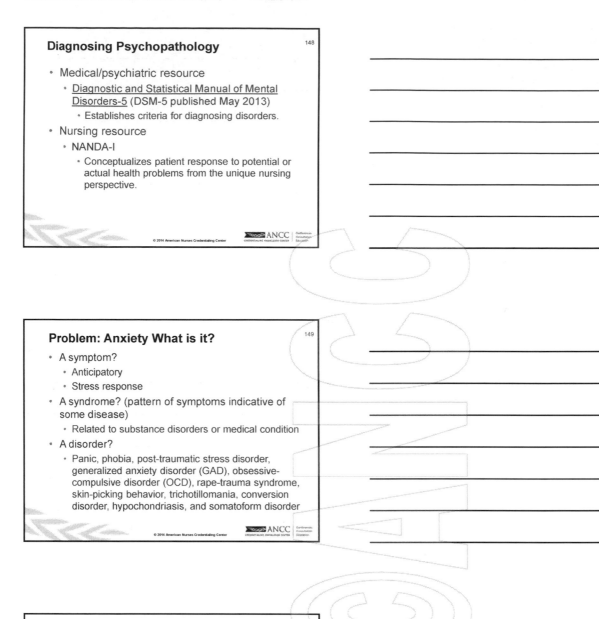

Diagnosing Psychopathology

148

- Medical/psychiatric resource
  - Diagnostic and Statistical Manual of Mental Disorders-5 (DSM-5 published May 2013)
    - Establishes criteria for diagnosing disorders.
- Nursing resource
  - NANDA-I
    - Conceptualizes patient response to potential or actual health problems from the unique nursing perspective.

© 2014 American Nurses Credentialing Center

Problem: Anxiety What is it?

149

- A symptom?
  - Anticipatory
  - Stress response
- A syndrome? (pattern of symptoms indicative of some disease)
  - Related to substance disorders or medical condition
- A disorder?
  - Panic, phobia, post-traumatic stress disorder, generalized anxiety disorder (GAD), obsessive-compulsive disorder (OCD), rape-trauma syndrome, skin-picking behavior, trichotillomania, conversion disorder, hypochondriasis, and somatoform disorder

© 2014 American Nurses Credentialing Center

Anxiety and Anxiety Disorders: Biology

150

- ANS sympathetic division activation
  - Peripheral fight/flight noradrenergic (NE) symptoms
    - Increased heart rate, respiratory rate, skin sweat, tremor, and pupil dilation.
- HPA axis activation
  - **Hypothalamus** secretes CRH.
  - CRH stimulates **pituitary** to release ACTH.
  - ACTH stimulates **adrenal** gland to release cortisol (glucocorticoids).
- Neurotransmitter alterations
  - GABA, NE, E

© 2014 American Nurses Credentialing Center

Anxiety and Anxiety Disorders: Psychological and Emotional

151

- Emotions associated with activation of the stress response systems are fear and anxiety.
  - Serotonin and GABA involved in suppressing the fear circuit.

- Medications used to treat anxiety disorders act directly at the level of the amygdala to suppress the fear circuit.
  - SSRIs increase serotonin.
  - Benzodiazepines increase GABA.

© 2014 American Nurses Credentialing Center

Anxiety Disorders Across the Life Span

152

Failure to Thrive (FTT)
- Infantile depression?

Separation Anxiety Disorder
- Separation anxiety is a normal stage of development around 6 to 18 months
- In childhood, continued fear of separation causes significant impairment.

Generalized Anxiety Disorder (GAD)
- Worry wart children - more frequent in females
- Average age of onset is in the 20s

Obsessive-Compulsive Disorder (OCD)
- Onset can occur before age 9
- High comorbidity with ADHD and tics

Panic Disorder
- Can present before puberty, though peak age 15 to 20

Phobias and PTSD
- Requires exposure to a fearful or threatening event

© 2014 American Nurses Credentialing Center

Risk Factors for Anxiety Disorders

153

- Genetics
- Biological
  - Temperament, physiologic abnormalities
- Medical conditions
  - For example, acute MI, or hypoglycemia
- Psychoanalytic
  - Unconscious fear expressed symbolically
  - Lack of ego-strength and coping resources
- Learning theory
  - Fears are learned and become conditioned responses.
  - Lack of recovery environment (social supports)
- Cognitive theory
  - Faulty cognitions or anxiety-inducing self instructions

© 2014 American Nurses Credentialing Center

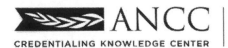

NANDA-I: Anxiety and Anxiety Disorders 154

- Panic anxiety: Real or perceived threat
- Powerlessness related to anxiety
- Ineffective coping related to intrusive or inappropriate thoughts
- Ineffective role performance related to ritual performance
- Post-trauma syndrome related to war exposure
- Post-traumatic rape syndrome related to sexual abuse, assault, or molestation
- Dysfunctional grieving
- Fear
- Social isolation

© 2014 American Nurses Credentialing Center

Problem: Psychotic (Thought) Disorders 155

- Genetic/Neurodevelopmental (prenatal period)
  - Brain abnormalities: Migrational defects, excessive, inadequate, or improper pruning of neurons/synapses.
  - Possible exposure to early virus or other insult
  - Smaller frontal and temporal lobes with enlarged ventricles.
- Biologic/Biochemical: Neurotransmitters
  - Positive and negative symptoms resulting from dopamine excess in mesolimbic brain pathway.
  - Excitotoxic death (neurodegeneration) of neurons.

© 2014 American Nurses Credentialing Center

Risk Factors for Psychotic (Thought) Disorders 156

- Environmental
  - Stress-Diathesis Theory
  - Infection and birth season

- Medical
  - Substance intoxication or withdrawal
  - Epilepsy
  - Organic and cognitive impairments (dementia, delirium)

© 2014 American Nurses Credentialing Center

4 Phases of Schizophrenia 157

1. Prodromal Phase: Onset lasts days to years
   - Functional deterioration; this may include substance abuse.
   - Goals: Minimize stress, enhance adaptation, continued symptom reduction, and functional recovery.
   - Treatment: Remain on antipsychotic at least six months.
2. Acute Phase: can last one to six months.
   - Positive and Negative symptoms:
     - Positive: Delusions, hallucinations, disorganized speech, and disorganized or catatonic behavior
     - Negative: Alogia, avolition, anhedonia, and affective flattening
   - Onset: Males: 18 to 25 years; Females: 25 to 35 years.
   - Goals: Prevent harm, control disturbed behavior, reduce positive symptoms, return to best level of functioning, alliance with patient and family, form short- and long-term goals, and community and support referrals.
   - Treatment: First-line - Atypical antipsychotics.

© 2014 American Nurses Credentialing Center

4 Phases of Schizophrenia (cont.) 158

3. Stabilization or Recovery Phase: May take several months
   - Impairment characterized by negative symptoms
   - Goals: Minimize stress, enhance adaptation, continued symptom reduction, and functional recovery
   - Treatment: Remain on antipsychotic at least six months.
4. Residual or Maintenance Phase: SPMI=severely and persistently mentally ill.
   - Some degree of persisting impairment remains .
   - Goals: Ensure that symptom remission or control is sustained; maintain or improve level of functioning and quality of life; treat increases in symptoms or relapses; continue to monitor for adverse effects.
   - Treatments: Assess for AIMs, metabolic syndrome, EPS, blood glucose, and psychosocial support. Antipsychotic meds can reduce risk of relapse to less than 30% per year.

© 2014 American Nurses Credentialing Center

NANDA: Schizophrenia and Schizoaffective Disorder 159

- Disturbed thought processes related to
  - Delusional thoughts
- Disturbed sensory perceptions related to
  - Auditory hallucinations
- Social isolation related to
  - Mistrust of others
  - Withdrawal
- Risk for violence to self or others related to
  - Rage reactions, anxiety
- Impaired verbal communication related to
  - Regression or anxiety
  - Disordered thought processes

© 2014 American Nurses Credentialing Center

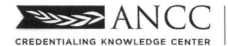
Review Question
160

* During admission interview, a 45 year old admitted 3 days ago with major depressive disorder hangs her head, starts wringing her hands rapidly, cries aloud and reports an experience of nonconsensual molestation in the last week? What is an appropriate nursing diagnosis for this patient?

a) Sexual dysfunction
b) Complicated grieving
c) Rape trauma syndrome
d) Ineffective self health management

© 2014 American Nurses Credentialing Center

Review Question
161

* Mr. Folly, age 54, a homeless man has been readmitted to the inpatient psychiatric unit 4 times in the past 4 months. He is well known to psychiatric services, and today he is begging for admission because "I hurt. I need medicine. I am suicidal and I mean it." His past psychiatric history is positive for major depressive disorder, HIV/AIDS, post hip replacement 6 months ago at the VA hospital. He shows nurse 2 empty bottles of Vicodin and 1 empty bottle of Truvada (antiviral). He states that he takes Vicodin 4 times a day and Truvada once a day. PE reveals the following:

* CD4 count 143; no allergies; BP 188/102; P 124; R 26; T 101. What is the nurse's priority concern for the patient? Patient may be:

A. In narcotic withdrawal
B. Exhibiting full-blown AIDS dementia
C. Exhibiting post-operative infection
D. Experiencing somatic delusions and needing support.

© 2014 American Nurses Credentialing Center

003: The Nursing Process in Psychiatric Nursing: Diagnosis & Planning (Part 2)

ANCC

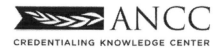
003: Learning Objectives (Part 2)

163

1. Discuss appropriate care plans utilizing evidence-based strategies and therapeutic environments for improved patient outcomes.
2. Identify nurse-initiated and collaborative (e.g., interprofessional) strategies for improved patient outcomes.

© 2014 American Nurses Credentialing Center

Problem: Mood Disorders

164

* Disruptive Mood Disorder Dysregulation (DMDD): Major Depression
* Dysthymia
* Bipolar I
* Bipolar II
* Adjustment disorder

© 2014 American Nurses Credentialing Center

Mood Disorders Across the Life Span

165

* Self-Mutilation
  * Are tattoos a socially acceptable mask for SM?
* Average age of onset
  * Bipolar Disorder
    * Childhood (5 to 6 years) to age 50
    * Mean age of onset: Age 21 to 30
  * Major depressive disorder
    * Can occur at any age
    * Generally between ages 20 and 50
    * Mean age of onset: Age 40
  * Early onset may be triggered by significant stressors

© 2014 American Nurses Credentialing Center

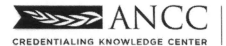
Depression: Biochemical and Physiological Theories

166

* Monoamine Hypothesis:
  * Deficits in the monoamine systems (serotonin, norepinephrine, dopamine) that cause depression.
  * Evidence: All antidepressants increase one or more of the monoamines, hence reduce symptoms.

* Vitamin D_3 deficiency theory:
  * Evidence suggests Vitamin D has beneficial neurological effects on cognition, memory, and mood*.

* (Farrington, 2013)

© 2014 American Nurses Credentialing Center

Depression: HPA Axis Dysregulation

167

* The HPA axis: Main site where genetic and environmental influences converge to cause mood disorders.
* Feedback loop: Hypothalamus (CRH) to anterior pituitary gland (ACTH) to adrenal gland (cortisol).
* Evidence
  * Individuals with major depressive disorder often present with hypercortisolemia, resistance of cortisol to suppression by dexamethasone, blunted ACTH responses to CRH challenge, and elevated CRH concentrations in the CSF.

© 2014 American Nurses Credentialing Center

Risk Factors for Mood Disorders

168

* Genetic

* Environmental
  * Stress–Diathesis Theory
    * Childhood loss or trauma
    * Stressful life events

* Medical or Biologic
  * Co-morbid with other illnesses
    * Cardiovascular disease, stroke, Parkinson's, cognitive dysfunction, anxiety disorder, traumatic brain injury, hypothyroidism, or cancer.

© 2014 American Nurses Credentialing Center

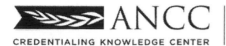
Symptoms of Depression

169

Affective
- Hopelessness
- Worthlessness and despair
- Apathy and anhedonia
- Emptiness

Behavioral
- Psychomotor retardation or agitation
- Verbal communication decreased
- Hygiene and grooming decreased
- Social isolation
- Anhedonia

Cognitive
- Confusion
- Indecisiveness
- Concentration decreased
- Self blame
- Suicidal ideation

Physical
- Body slowdown
- Sleep disturbances
- Vegetative symptoms (change in sleep and appetite)

© 2014 American Nurses Credentialing Center

NANDA-I: Major Depression

170

- Risk for suicide related to:
  - Feelings of hopelessness, helplessness, or worthlessness
  - Anger turned inwards
  - Reality distortions.
- Low self-esteem related to:
  - Learned helplessness
  - Significant losses
  - Cognitive distortions of negative self image.

- Dysfunctional grieving related to:
  - Real or perceived loss
  - Bereavement overload (not adequately dealing with losses)>
- Social isolation related to:
  - Negative self perception
  - Egocentric behaviors.

© 2014 American Nurses Credentialing Center

Symptoms of Bipolar Disorders

171

- Expansive, cheerful mood
- Irritable when wishes unfulfilled
- Flighty, rapid flow of ideas
- Increased behavior
- Lack depth of personality and warmth
- Increased libido or sexual promiscuity
- Irresponsible financial management
- Loquacious (more talkative than usual)

- Continuous high elation
- Emotional lability: Rapid changes
- Fragmented, racing, and disjointed thoughts
- Extreme hyperactivity
- Delusions, hallucinations
- Increased, disorganized, and incoherent speech
- Flamboyant dress
- Grandiosity and inflated sense of self

Onset: between ages 15 and 30.

© 2014 American Nurses Credentialing Center

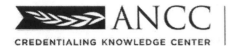
NANDA-I: Bipolar Disorders

172

- Risk for injury related to…
- Risk for violence (self or other directed) related to…
- Disturbed thought processes related to…
- Disturbed sensory perception related to…
- Nutritional deficiency related to…
- Impaired social interaction related to…

© 2014 American Nurses Credentialing Center

Personality and Personality Disorders

173

- Personality
  - Temperamental traits are present at birth,
  - Personality forms during childhood: Influenced by attachment, parenting style, experiences.
  - Enduring characteristics present by late adolescence.
- Personality Disorder
  - Onset in adolescence or early adulthood
- Personality changes (pathophysiology not well understood)
  - AIDS, dementia, drug abuse

© 2014 American Nurses Credentialing Center

General Criteria for Personality Disorders

174

- Enduring pattern of inner experience and behavior.
- Manifested in two or more of the following:
  - Cognition (ways of perceiving and interpreting self, other people, and events)
  - Affectivity (range, intensity, lability, and appropriateness of emotional response)
  - Interpersonal functioning
  - Impulse control problems.
- Pattern is inflexible, stable, and pervasive (long duration).
- Clinically significant distress or impairment.
- Onset traced back at least to adolescence or early adulthood.
- Not better accounted for by another mental disorder.
- Not due to substance or medical condition.

© 2014 American Nurses Credentialing Center

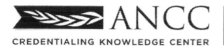
Risk Factors for Personality Disorders

175

- Genetics
- Developmental
  - Behavior pattern in childhood or early adolescence in which the rights of others or age-appropriate norms are violated
  - Lack of empathy
  - Low level of fear
  - May be a precursor to Antisocial Personality Disorder which is diagnosed after age 18 and up.
- Sociocultural and familial
  - Prenatal exposure to noxious chemicals
  - Physical abuse history

Personality Disorders: 3 Clusters

176

- Cluster A (odd, eccentric, loner, ESP types):
  1. Paranoid PD
  2. Schizotypal PD
  3. Schizoid PD

- Cluster B: (cunning, users, con men, erratic, dramatic, self-absorbed types):
  1. Antisocial PD
  2. Borderline PD
  3. Histrionic PD
  4. Narcissistic PD

- Cluster C (timid, needy, "intentional/unintentional" failures types):
  1. Obsessive-Compulsive PD
  2. Dependent PD
  3. Avoidant PD

Problem: Cluster A Personality Disorders

177

1. Paranoid PD: Suspicious, mistrustful, defensive or resistant to control; skeptical of most things; copes using projection (attributes one's shortcomings to others to feel justified in their actions).
   - Therapeutic approach
     - Help patient to develop trust and intimacy; overzealous use of interpretation increases patients' mistrust significantly.
2. Schizoid PD: Asocial pattern, aloof, introverted, seclusive, uninterested in social activities, apathetic, unengaged, may be schizophrenia prodrome, copes using intellectualization.
   - Therapeutic approach
     - Encourage social activity, use role playing, and/or homework.

Problem: Cluster A Personality Disorders (cont.) 178

3. Schizotypal PD: Odd, bizarre, strange, magical, eccentric, socially anxious, secretive and private, copes using undoing; easily overwhelmed by stimulation. Many bizarre acts/thoughts reflect a retraction of previous acts/thoughts.
   - Therapeutic approach
     - Provide behavioral intervention through social skills training
     - Trust is important.

© 2014 American Nurses Credentialing Center

Problem: Cluster B Personality Disorders 179

1. Antisocial PD: Psychopath, delinquent or criminal, lack of superego, impulsive, thrill seeking, irresponsible, gets pleasure from swindling others and copes by acting out.
   - Therapeutic approach
     - Therapy is usually an ultimatum. Patient will try to form alliance against others or con therapist. Cognitive Behavioral Therapy (CBT) helps to point out how adopted behaviors may be disadvantageous in long run.
     - Therapeutic Communities (Maxwell Jones) offers participatory and highly structured group-based rehabilitation residential settings based on milieu therapies.
       - Example: Another Way Transitional Living Program in New Hampshire provides supportive housing using professionals and peers to help individuals transition from substance use to improved health.

© 2014 American Nurses Credentialing Center

Problem: Cluster B Personality Disorders (cont.) 180

2. Borderline PD: Unstable, intense affect, impulsive, identity disturbance, chaotic relationships, manipulative, abandonment concerns, demanding, unpredictable, "black or white", "all or nothing" thinking, copes using regression, projection, and denial.
   - Therapeutic approach
     - Teach patient to talk about feelings instead of acting.
     - Teach patient to tolerate feelings. Analyze countertransference reactions. Limit-setting and boundaries are important. CBT deals with negative thinking; Dialectical Behavioral Therapy (DBT) is a type of CBT that helps with dealing with issues of suicidality and self-harm; focuses on acceptance and validation of the self.

© 2014 American Nurses Credentialing Center

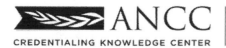

Problem: Cluster B Personality Disorders 181
(cont.)

3. Histrionic PD: Gregarious; seductive; dramatic; tendency to sexualize all relationships, extreme extraversion, attention seeking; superficial; difficulty in maintaining deep relationships; copes by creating facades.
   - Therapeutic approach
     - Set specific goals. Help patient to define a personal identity Teach to think instead of to feel.

© 2014 American Nurses Credentialing Center

Problem: Cluster B Personality 182
Disorders

4. Narcissistic PD: Egotistical; preoccupied with power and prestige; sense of superiority; arrogant, entitled; and copes using rationalization, repression, fantasy.
   - Therapeutic approach
     - Teach that imperfections are not a sign of failure, help patient accept a realistic self image. Set limits d/t testing behaviors. Patient will usually try to devalue therapist through superiority stance.

© 2014 American Nurses Credentialing Center

Problem: Cluster C Personality 183
Disorders

1. Avoidant PD: Sensitive to rejection/humiliation, withdrawn, slow and constrained speech, shy and uncomfortable with others, sees self as inferior, copes using fantasy and daydreams.
   - Therapeutic approach
     - Support before confrontation, diminish anticipation of pain, decrease sensitivity, and help to improve self-image.

© 2014 American Nurses Credentialing Center

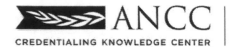
Problem: Cluster C Personality Disorders (cont.)

184

2. Dependent PD: Submissive, needs social approval, clingy, feels inadequate, wants other to manage their lives, relates to others in an immature/child-like way, naïve, copes using introjection (internalizes others' beliefs).

   - Therapeutic approach
     - Don't reinforce patient's desire to become dependent on you. Is patient's apparent improvement just a search for approval?

Problem: Cluster C Personality Disorders (cont.)

185

3. Obsessive-Compulsive PD: Conforming, meticulous, rigid, disciplined, concerned with order and conformity, stubborn, usually copes using reaction-formation (doing the opposite of their feelings), isolation, and undoing.

   - Therapeutic approach
     - Cognitive Behavioral Therapy (CBT): Type of therapy used in conjunction with medications.

Substance Use Disorder (SUD)

186

- A problematic pattern of substance use leading to significant impairment with at least two criteria in a 12 month period (DSM-5).

- Criteria rated as
  - Mild: 2-3 criteria
  - Moderate: 4-5 criteria
  - Severe: 6 or more criteria
  - Craving: A new criteria for assessment and treatment.

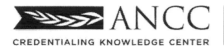

Risk Factors for Substance Use Disorders 187

- Biology/Genetics
  - Biochemical/neuroanatomical brain alterations from chronic use may influence vulnerability and promote addiction.
    - Drugs derive their rewarding properties from altering dopamine levels in limbic system triggering cravings.
    - Dopamine in the brain mediates pleasure/motivation.
- Psychological/Mental Illness
  - Low self-esteem, frequent depression, or passivity.
  - Inability to relax or defer gratification.
  - Higher risk in impulsive groups: Violent offenders, conduct disorder, intermittent explosive disorder.
- Sociocultural
  - Social learning (e.g., cultural, ethnic, peer influences), conditioning.
  - Stress increases alcohol and drug use and is associated with higher rates of relapse.

© 2014 American Nurses Credentialing Center

Substance Abuse and Mental Illness Are Linked 100

- SA and MI share risk and protective factors
  - Up to half with a serious mental illness will develop a substance use disorder at some time in their lives.
  - Substance users are almost 3x's as likely to have a serious mental illness as those who do not have a substance use disorder.
  - 3 in 4 mental illnesses emerge early in life and 1 in 5 children have had a serious mental illness.
- "A chronic, relapsing, disease of the brain that has imbedded behavioral and social context aspects." (A. Leohnor, 1998, former head of NIDA)

© 2014 American Nurses Credentialing Center

Substance Intoxication and Withdrawal 180

- Intoxication: Substance-specific syndrome
  - Reversible syndrome caused by substance ingestion.
  - Maladaptive behaviors due to substances.
  - Symptoms not due to medical conditions or other mental disorder.
- Withdrawal: Substance-specific syndrome
  - Caused by cessation of prolonged and heavy use.
  - Causing impairment in social, occupational, and other areas of functioning.
- Withdrawal symptoms are generally the opposite of intoxication symptoms. Symptoms not due to, or accounted to other mental disorder.

© 2014 American Nurses Credentialing Center

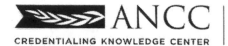
Substance Dependence 190

- Physical Dependence
  - Physiologic state of neuro-adaptation produced by repeated administration of a drug, necessitating continued administration to prevent withdrawal syndrome.
  - Substance often is taken in larger amounts or over a longer period than intended to achieve desired effect (tolerance).
  - Cravings for the drug.
- Psychological Dependence
  - Repeats use to produce pleasure or avoid discomfort.
  - Obsessions and compulsions: Thought and time spent in activities to obtain the substance.
  - Social, occupational, and recreational activities given up.
  - Unsuccessful efforts to cut down use.
  - Substance abuse results in more deaths, illnesses, and disabilities than any other preventable condition.

Problem: Alcohol and the Brain 191

- Enhances GABA
- Evidence of:
  - Less brain growth and more brain shrinkage (amount of shrinkage increases with age)
  - Enlarged brain sulci, fissures, and ventricles from loss of gray and white matter
  - Affected structures include the prefrontal cortex (executive functioning) and the hippocampus (memory).
- Alcohol ingestion via new routes - Smoking vapors, rectal instillations bypasses CYP450 first pass system; direct to bloodstream.

Problem: Alcohol 192

Assess current symptoms and history:
- Intoxicated: CNS depression or agitation, and motor impairment.
- Withdrawal: Anxiety, tremor, seizure, delirium, or death.

Screening
- CAGE, Brief Drug Abuse Screening Test (B-DAST)

- Behavioral and physical findings
  - Peripheral neuropathy, myopathy, or cardiomyopathy
  - Wernicke's encephalopathy, Korsakoff's psychosis
  - Esophagitis, pancreatitis, gastritis, hepatitis, or cirrhosis
  - Serum or urine analysis: Leukopenia, thrombocytopenia, increased GGT, AST, ALT, ALP, MCV, ammonia, amylase, or triglycerides
  - Sexual dysfunction
  - Jaundice

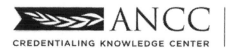
Problem: Sedative-Hypnotics and Anxiolytics

193

- CNS depressants enhance GABA:
  - Benzodiazepines (including midazolam [Versed]), barbiturates, alcohol, and propofol.
- Assessment
  - Cognitive slowing and/or memory problems,
  - Sedation and sleep,
  - Decreased anxiety or decreased musculoskeletal tension, and
  - Sexual dysfunction.
- Used to treat alcohol and other substance withdrawal; anticonvulsant, and anti-seizure effects.

© 2014 American Nurses Credentialing Center

Problem: Amphetamine and Other Stimulants

194

- CNS Stimulants: Increases both DA and N
  - Amphetamines, methamphetamines, Bath Salts, or Khat
  - Cocaine, caffeine, nicotine (non-amphetamine stimulant)
  - Some OTC (over-the-counter) medications
- Assessment
  - CNS: Initial euphoria may be followed by crashing; repeated use can lead to acute paranoid psychosis. Basal ganglia affects can cause increased stereotypic behaviors (pacing, scratching).
  - PNS: Tremor, emotional lability, or restlessness.
  - Cardiovascular/pulmonary: Tachycardia, ventricular irritability, respiratory depression
  - Gastrointestinal: Constipation
  - Renal: Urinary retention

© 2014 American Nurses Credentialing Center

Problem: Inhalants

195

- "Huffing" substances
  - Gasoline or varnish remover
  - Lighter fluid
  - Glue, spray paint
- Assessment
  - Psychological: Belligerent, assaultive, apathy, impaired judgment, psychosis.
  - Physical: Dizziness, Nystagmus, incoordination, slurred speech, unsteady gait, depressed reflexes, tremor, blurred vision, euphoria, or anorexia.
- Withdrawal similar to alcohol.

© 2014 American Nurses Credentialing Center

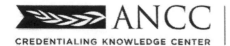
Problem: Opioids

196

- CNS depressants (narcotics, analgesics)
  - Morphine, codeine, dilaudid, methadone, demerol; Vicodin and Oxycodone are the most commonly abused legal drugs.
  - Heroin is the most commonly abused illegal drug.
- Assessment
  - CNS: Pain relief, euphoria (rush), tranquility, drowsiness (nodding), mood swings, mental clouding, apathy, constricted pupils.
  - PNS: Slowed motor movements.
  - Respiratory depression – major cause of death.
- Withdrawal
  - Drug craving, lacrimation, rhinorrhea, yawning, diaphoresis, and/or flu-like symptoms.
  - Scale: Clinical Opioid Withdrawal Scale (COWS).

© 2014 American Nurses Credentialing Center
ANCC

Problem: Hallucinogens

197

- Psychedelic substances: interfere with glutamate functioning
  - Mescaline and/or psilocybin
  - LSD and/or STP
  - Phencyclidine (PCP): anesthetic
  - Designer drugs (Ecstasy; Molly's; Special K or Ketamine)
    - Ecstasy is neurotoxic to serotonin and its cells
- Assessment
  - CNS: "Trips" (changes in sensory experience, including illusions, and hallucinations), impaired judgment, fear of losing one's mind, anxiety, or delirium
  - PNS: Heightened sensory awareness, staggering gait, or slurred speech
  - Cardiovascular: Tachycardia, increased BP, or hyperthermia
  - GI: Nausea
- Withdrawal: Flashbacks?

© 2014 American Nurses Credentialing Center
ANCC

Problem: Cannabis

198

- Substances:
  - Marijuana (active ingredient is THC: Tetrahydrocannabinol)
  - K2 (Spice): Synthetic marijuana
  - Hashish
- Assessment:
  - CNS: Can have both stimulant and sedative properties, well-being, relaxation, loss of temporal awareness, slowing of thought processes, shortened attention span, easy distractibility, impairment of short-term memory (hippocampal damage), apathy, panic, toxic delirium; and sometimes psychosis
  - GI: Increased appetite or anti-nausea
- Withdrawal:
  - Difficulty sleeping or irritability

© 2014 American Nurses Credentialing Center
ANCC

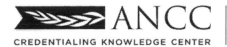

Problem: Nicotine (Tobacco)

199

- CNS stimulant
- Induces liver enzymes
- Relieves negative symptoms of schizophrenia.
- Highly addictive
- Approx. 70-85% people diagnosed with a mental illness use nicotine
- Clinical scale to measure withdrawal
  - Fagerstrom Test for Nicotine Dependence (smoker and smokeless versions)
- Popular today
  - Hookah bars: Flavored smokes
  - E-cigs

NANDA-I: Substance Use Disorders

200

- Impaired judgment
- Imbalanced nutrition
- Ineffective coping
- Risk of injury

Risk Factors for Eating Disorders

201

- Biological
  - Illnesses that cause changes in appetite or weight
  - More common in females
- Sociocultural
  - Family dynamics
  - Cultural focus on being thin
- Psychological
  - Difficulties with growing up
  - Poor sexual adjustment or sexual trauma/abuse

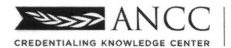
NANDA-I: Gender Dysphoria 202

- Disturbed body image
- Disturbed personal identity
- Risk for compromised human dignity
- Role confusion
- Depression
- Hopelessness

© 2014 American Nurses Credentialing Center

Problem: Anorexia Nervosa 203

- Body weight less than 85% of expected based on age and height
- Cachexia: Loss of fat, muscle mass, reduced thyroid metabolism, cold intolerance, and difficulty in maintaining core temperature
- Cardiac: Loss of muscle, arrhythmias, bradycardia, or tachycardia
- Dermatologic: Lanugo or edema
- Hematological: Leukopenia
- Skeletal: Osteoporosis

© 2014 American Nurses Credentialing Center

Problem: Bulimia 204

- Bulimia: Purging type
  - Metabolic disturbances related to vomiting, and laxative abuse
    - Electrolyte abnormalities: Hypokalemic, hypochloremic alkalosis, or hypomagnesaemia

- Bulimia: Non-purging type
  - Inappropriate compensatory behaviors may include fasting or excessive exercise, but not vomiting, laxatives, or enemas

© 2014 American Nurses Credentialing Center

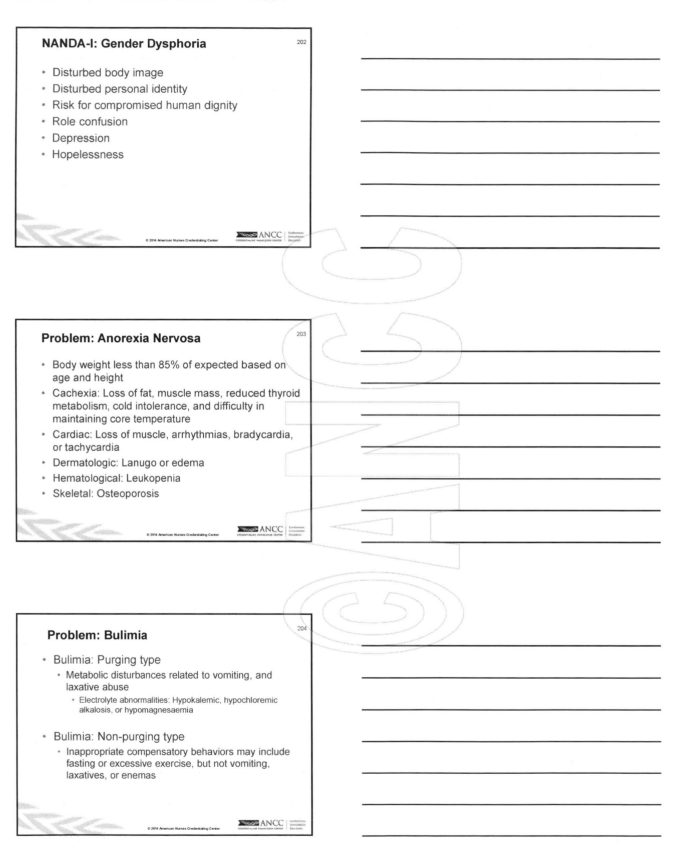

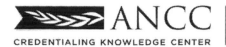
Problem: Binge Eating Disorder

205

- New to DSM5
- Recurring episodes of eating significantly more food in short period of time with feelings of lack of control
  - Eat quickly and uncontrollably despite feeling full
  - Feels guilt or shame or disgust afterwards
  - Eats alone
  - Less common, more severe than overeating
  - Associated with significant physical and psychological problems

Problem: Obesity

206

- Excess body fat
  - Prevalence of childhood obesity has doubled since 1980 in the U.S.
  - Hormonal causes: Hypothyroidism, hypercortisolism, primary hyperinsulinism, pseudohypoparathyroidism, acquired hypothalamic problems (e.g., tumors, infections, traumatic syndromes)
  - Complications
    - Lower metabolic rate from lack of exercise
    - Increased risk for other health problems including diabetes, hypertension, and premature heart disease

NANDA-I: Eating Disorders, including FTT and Geriatric Failure to Thrive (GTT)

207

- Risk for electrolyte or fluid imbalance
- Nutrition, altered, and less or more than body requirements
- Readiness for enhanced nutrition
- Risk for self-injury
- Self-care deficit or feeding
- Body image disturbance
- Ineffective coping
- Risk for impaired attachment
- Dysfunctional family processes

Problem: Dementia

208

- Cognitive disorder represented by progressive deterioration of mental activity and self care abilities; memory impairment and cognitive deficits are disabling and represents a decline from previous functioning; syndrome of intellectual impairment.

- Onset is slow and insidious.

- Score of 24/30 or less on the MMSE is suggestive of cognitive difficulties and should be confirmed with more extensive neuropsychological testing.

© 2014 American Nurses Credentialing Center — ANCC

Dementia Classifications

209

- Primary: Organic brain disease, for example Alzheimer's
  - Accounts for two-thirds of all dementias,
  - Age of onset: More common after age 65, and
  - Definitive diagnosis at autopsy.
- Secondary: Caused by other processes
  - Infection
  - Cerebrovascular accident; atherosclerosis
  - Neurosyphilis
  - Electrolyte (metabolic) imbalances
  - Drug toxicity
  - Sensory impairment (visual/auditory)
  - Emotional disturbances
  - Nutritional disturbances
  - Cerebral trauma or tumor
  - HIV

© 2014 American Nurses Credentialing Center — ANCC

Risk Factors for Dementia

210

- Neurotransmitter Dysfunction
  - Cholinergic deficit hypothesis
    - Evidence: Cholinesterase inhibitors boosts memory function in early dementia
  - Glutamate excitotoxicity leads to neurodegeneration
    - Evidence: Memantine (Namenda), blocks over-excitation of glutamate receptors; appears to stabilize degenerative course of Alzheimer Disease
- Neuronal Dysfunction:
  - Neurofibrillary tangles
    - Bundles of tangled proteins disrupt neuronal functioning
  - Neuritic plaques with beta-amyloid cores
    - Abnormal deposition of beta-amyloid destroys neurons

© 2014 American Nurses Credentialing Center — ANCC

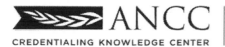
Progression of Alzheimer's Dementia

211

- Early
  - Forgetfulness and short-term memory loss
- Middle
  - Difficulty with familiar tasks such as cooking or balancing a checkbook
  - Changes in ability to communicate
  - Agnosia or apraxic
- Late
  - Inability to perform ADL's
  - Becomes disoriented, incoherent, amnesic, and/or incontinent

© 2014 American Nurses Credentialing Center

Progression of AIDS Dementia

212

- Early signs mimic depression
  - Hopelessness, insomnia, or forgetfulness
- Cognitive
  - Forgetfulness, slowness, poor concentration, and difficulties with problem-solving
- Behavioral
  - Apathy, social withdrawal
  - Possible delirium, delusions, or hallucinations
- Physical findings
  - Tremor, impaired rapid repetitive movements, imbalance, ataxia, hypertonia, hyperreflexia, frontal release signs, and/or CD4 depression

© 2011 American Nurses Credentialing Center

NANDA-I: Dementia

213

- Risk for injury
- Impaired verbal communication
- Self-care deficits (in bathing, hygiene, dressing, and grooming) related to cognitive impairment
- Disturbed social interactions
- Disturbed thought processes as evidenced by memory loss
- Disturbed sleep pattern
- Caregiver Role Strain

© 2011 American Nurses Credentialing Center

Problem: Delirium

214

- Cognitive disturbance in level of consciousness accompanied by a change in cognition that cannot be better accounted for by a preexisting or evolving dementia.
- Onset characteristics:
  - Cognition changes rapidly; acute confusion that fluctuates; psychomotor agitation or depression may be present
  - Often results directly from an underlying condition, such as a urinary tract infection
  - Reduced ability to maintain and shift attention.
- Occurs frequently in medical/rehabilitation settings; often unrecognized and can result in considerable morbidity and mortality.

© 2014 American Nurses Credentialing Center

Risk Factors for Delirium:

"I WATCH DEATH"

215

- **I**nfection (urinary tract infection)
- **W**ithdrawal (substance use or alcoholism)
- **A**cute metabolic disturbance
- **T**rauma
- **C**NS pathology (sensory impairment, history of delirium, or pre-existing dementia)
- **H**ypoxia
- **D**eficiencies (impaired liver function; malnutrition)
- **E**ndocrinopathies
- **A**cute vascular
- **T**oxins (multiple medications)
- **H**eavy metals

© 2014 American Nurses Credentialing Center

Child and Adolescent Disorders

216

- Anxiety
- Mood disorders
- Schizophrenia (rare)
- Pervasive Developmental Disorders (PDD)
- ADHD
- Eating disorders
- Oppositional Defiant Disorder (ODD)
- Conduct Disorder (CD)

- Pediatric Autoimmune Neuropsychiatric Disorder (PANDAS)
- Reactive Attachment Disorder (RAD)
- Adjustment Disorder
- Disruptive Mood Dysregulation Disorder (DMDD)
- Non-Suicidal Self Injury (NSSI)

BELIEVE REPORTS OF SEXUAL ABUSE, SEXUAL VIOLENCE, MOLESTATION

© 2014 American Nurses Credentialing Center

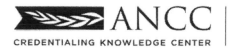
Problem: Neurodevelopmental Disorders

217

- Autism Spectrum Disorder
  - Affects one in 68 children (CDC, 3/2014)

  - Asperger's syndrome
    - Observed difficulties in social interactions and nonverbal communication
    - Cognitive and linguistic development intact

Problem: Neurodevelopmental Disorders

218

- Rett syndrome
  - Genetic mutation on X chromosome
  - Occurs only in girls. As she grows, she begins to lose purposeful use of hands and inability to speak; early problems crawling or walking
  - Can live until middle age. Silent Angels Story
- Childhood disintegrative disorder (aka Heller's Syndrome)
  - Apparent normal development to age 3, then regression in skills
  - Severe speech pathology

Risk Factors for Attention-Deficit Hyperactivity Disorder (ADHD)

219

- Two pathways mediate attention, arousal, concentration and related cognitive functions
  1. Norepinephrine prefrontal pathway
  2. Dopaminergic mesocortical/nigrostriatal pathway
- If they fail, symptoms may result.
- Evidence:
  - Increasing norepinephrine and dopamine with psychostimulants improves symptoms
  - In unaffected individuals, increasing dopamine with stimulants increases motor behavior and impulsivity, whereas patients with ADHD exhibit a paradoxical reduction

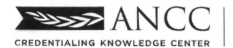
Problem: Attention-Deficit Hyperactivity Disorder (ADHD)

220

- Symptoms present before age 7
- Possible etiology contributors
  - Genetics
  - Perinatal complications
  - Neurological illness
  - Diet
  - Allergy
  - Environmental toxins
- Difficult to distinguish from early bipolar mania

© 2014 American Nurses Credentialing Center

Problem: ADHD: 3 Subtypes

221

Attention-Deficit Type

- Fails to pay close attention to detail
- Has difficulty sustaining attention
- Does not seem to listen
- Does not follow through
- Has difficulty organizing
- Avoids, dislikes, or is reluctant to engage in tasks that require sustained mental effort
- Loses things necessary for tasks
- Easily distracted
- Forgetful in daily activities

Hyperactive Type

- Leaves seat when sitting is expected
- Fidgets with hands or feet
- Runs about or climbs excessively
- Has difficulty playing quietly
- On the go
- Talks excessively

Impulsive Type

- Has difficulty waiting for turn
- Blurts out answers before questions are completed
- Interrupts or intrudes on others

© 2014 American Nurses Credentialing Center

Problem: PANDAS

222

- Pediatric Autoimmune Neuropsychiatric Disorder
  - Possibly an autoimmune disorder that affects the basal ganglia similar to Sydenham's Chorea.
- Onset of an Obsessive-Compulsive Disorder (OCD) or a tic disorder between the ages of 3 years and the beginning of puberty with the following:
  - Onset or exacerbation of symptoms related to infection with group A β-hemolytic streptococcus (GABHS infection)
  - Abrupt symptom onset; dramatic exacerbations
  - Neurologic abnormalities, hyperactivity, or choreiform movements.

© 2014 American Nurses Credentialing Center

Problem: Reactive Attachment Disorder

223

- Child fails to form normal attachments to primary caregivers in early childhood, poor bonding, poor attachment.
- May result from separation from caregivers between the ages of 6 months and 3 years, frequent change in caregivers lack of caregiver responsiveness.
  - (Children in orphanages; foster care situations where instability of living arrangements are available).
- Interpersonal and behavioral difficulties may occur later in life.

Problem: Adjustment Disorder

224

- Inability to cope with major life event.
- Sometimes referred to as a situational stressor.
  - Parents divorce, relocation/school change, failed grade in school, fired from job/retirement, job change, loss of significant other (boyfriend/girlfriend, spouse, etc.), loss of driving privileges
- May be acute or chronic.
- Resilience: Capacity to respond successfully to stressors, ability to "bounce back" adjust.
  - Explains why stressors do not affect everyone the same.

Problem: Disruptive Disorder

225

- Oppositional Defiance Disorder (ODD)
  - Symptoms of disruptive behavior patterns seen before age 8.
  - Characterized by:
    - Negativity
    - Defiance
    - Hostility toward authority
    - Blames others.

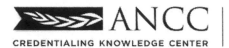
NANDA-I: Childhood Disorders, General

226

- Risk for self-directed violence
- Risk for other-directed violence
- Ineffective coping
  - Enuresis or encopresis
- Problems with social skills, problem solving, school performance
- Disturbed thought processes
- Disturbed sleep patterns
- Anxiety
- Chronic or situational low self-esteem
- Risk for caregiver role strain
- Readiness for enhanced family processes

NANDA-I: Family-Related

227

- Caregiver role strain
- Ineffective parenting
- Ineffective family coping
- Complicated grieving
- Ineffective therapeutic regime

Review Question

228

The following instructions are given following an appointment at the mental health clinic: (1) Complete elements of the Iowa Conners rating and return at next appointment for review, (2) complete a 7-day diary of all foods and fluids ingested for review, (3) Rate quality of interpersonal patterns. The patient is likely undergoing work-up and evaluation for:

a) Obesity
b) Alzheimer's
c) Bipolar Disorder
d) Attention-Deficit Hyperactivity Disorder

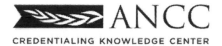
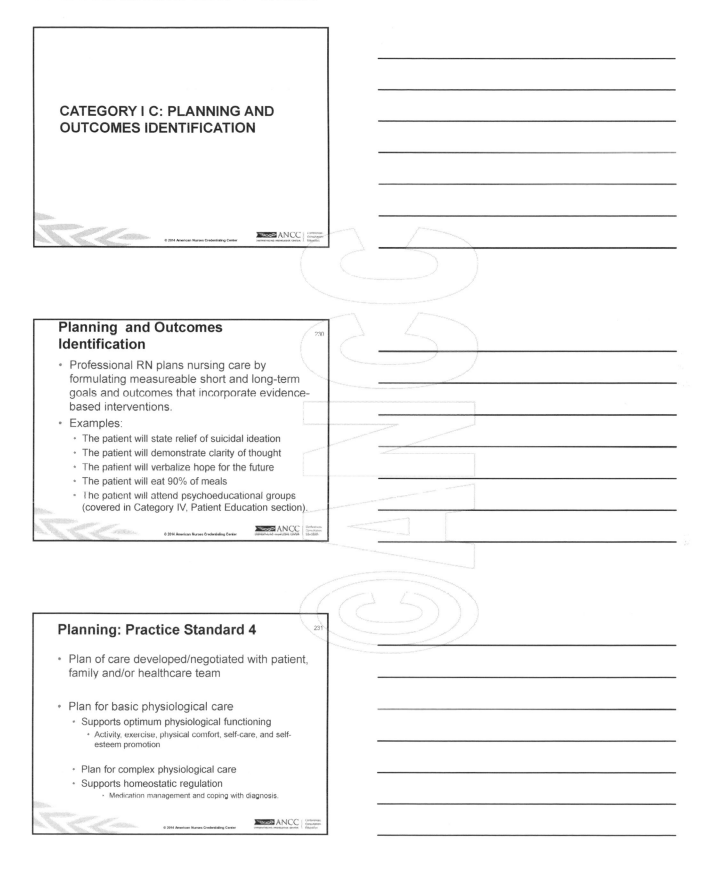

CATEGORY I C: PLANNING AND OUTCOMES IDENTIFICATION

© 2014 American Nurses Credentialing Center

Planning and Outcomes Identification

- Professional RN plans nursing care by formulating measureable short and long-term goals and outcomes that incorporate evidence-based interventions.
- Examples:
  - The patient will state relief of suicidal ideation
  - The patient will demonstrate clarity of thought
  - The patient will verbalize hope for the future
  - The patient will eat 90% of meals
  - The patient will attend psychoeducational groups (covered in Category IV, Patient Education section).

© 2014 American Nurses Credentialing Center

Planning: Practice Standard 4

- Plan of care developed/negotiated with patient, family and/or healthcare team

- Plan for basic physiological care
  - Supports optimum physiological functioning
    - Activity, exercise, physical comfort, self-care, and self-esteem promotion

  - Plan for complex physiological care
  - Supports homeostatic regulation
    - Medication management and coping with diagnosis.

© 2014 American Nurses Credentialing Center

Planning: Safety Risks Across the Life Span
232

Primary prevention: Parent education, school-based programs, education programs for older adults and caregivers, etc.

Infants
- Choking
- SIDS
- Falling
- Drowning
- Car accidents

Early childhood
- Drowning
- Pedestrian accidents
- Sharp objects
- Poisoning
- Falls
- Getting stuck in play objects (trunk, refrigerator)

School age
- Equipment accidents
- Bicycle injuries
- Sport injuries
- Electrical injuries
- Firearms

Adolescents
- Motor vehicle accidents
- Binge-drinking
- Sexually transmitted diseases
- Drug experimentation

Older adults
- Falls
- Accidents

© 2014 American Nurses Credentialing Center

Planning for Safety first! A High Priority
233

- TJC standards
  - Sentinel Events: Inpatient Suicide Recommendations for Prevention
- National Patient Safety Goals for 2014
  - Identify individuals served safety risks: Find out which individuals served are most likely to try to commit suicide.

© 2014 American Nurses Credentialing Center

Milieu Therapy: Practice Standard 5C
234

- Professional RN provides and structures the therapeutic environment in collaboration with patient and interdisciplinary team.
  - Safety provision
  - Community meetings

- The milieu is the environment or setting in which the treatment occurs.
  - Can be therapeutic or non-therapeutic.
  - Healthcare providers assess the environment to assure promotion of recovery and functionality.
  - If not therapeutic, nurse recommends changes to produce an appropriate setting.

© 2014 American Nurses Credentialing Center

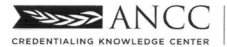
Therapeutic Milieu Settings

235

- Short-term inpatient treatment
- Community-based outpatient treatment
- Social service agencies including shelters and soup kitchens
- Healthcare clinics
- Church-sponsored activities
- Halfway and residential houses
- Correctional institutions
- Therapeutic communities

© 2014 American Nurses Credentialing Center

Planning Effective Environments

236

- Components
  - Safety
  - Structure
  - Norms
  - Limit-setting
  - Balance
  - Environmental modification: Milieu Therapy

© 2014 American Nurses Credentialing Center

Structural Issues

237

- Comfort during treatment
- Confidentiality of sensitive information
- Organization of healthful activities
- Structuring time and monitoring fatigue in both patients and staff
- Cleanliness of environment
- Access to communication
- Provision of space for privacy
- Provision of space when needed

© 2014 American Nurses Credentialing Center

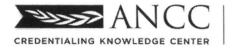
Norms: Expectations 238

- Community rules should be posted or accessible
- Consequences discussed before actions occur
- Violence, aggression, abuse prohibited
- Respect shown for patient, family, and staff
- Independence encouraged
- Communication safeguarded communication
- Cultural differences accepted
- Feedback promoted if positive
- Visitors monitored

© 2014 American Nurses Credentialing Center

Limit-Setting 239

- Behavior Modification
  - Limits set appropriately. No power plays.
  - Staff enforces rules consistently.
  - Individual uniqueness and needs considered.
  - Time-out opportunities offered.
  - Crisis intervention implemented.
  - Advocacy promoted.
  - One-on-one observation available.
  - Seclusion and restraints: last resort.
  - Medications as prescribed.
  - Token economy implemented:
    - Interpersonal skills and self-care behaviors rewarded.
    - Positive and negative reinforcement used.

© 2014 American Nurses Credentialing Center

Balance 240

- "Balance is the process of gradually allowing independent behaviors in a dependent situation" (Keltner, Schwecke, Bostrom, in Psychiatric Nursing, 4th edition, 2003, p 280-281).

- Independence needs to be gained in increments.

- Staff monitors that one's need does not overpower another's need, both in and between clients.

© 2014 American Nurses Credentialing Center

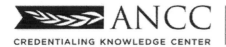

Environmental Modification 241

- Modification results from continual evaluation of effectiveness.

- Rules can change in accordance to the makeup and diagnoses of clients (sometimes there are grey areas).

- Clear communication is vital in all milieus in order to enhance effectiveness and promote recovery.

Outcomes: Basis for Evaluating Care 242

- Clinical outcomes
  - Health status, relapse, recurrence, readmission, number of episodes, symptomatology, coping responses, high risk behaviors, and incidence reports.
- Functional outcomes
  - Functional status (e.g., GAF), social interaction, ADLs, occupational abilities, quality of life, family relationships, and housing arrangements.
- Satisfaction outcomes
  - Satisfaction with treatment, treatment outcome and treatment team/organization, and patient satisfaction measures.
- Financial outcomes
  - Cost, revenue, length of stay, and use of resources.

Outcomes Identification Guidelines 243

- Patient and Family-Centered: Focuses on diagnosis; suited to patient or population of interest
- Singular: Separate goals for each identified problem or need
- Mutual: Agreed upon by patient/family and nurse/team/health care providers
- Measurable, reliable, valid: Describes quality, quantity, severity, frequency (standardized assessment tools and scales)
- Time-limited: short and long-term goals
- Realistic: Attainable to provide a sense of accomplishment; sensitive to changes within or across individuals
- Evidence-based: Algorithms, Practice Guidelines, Clinical Pathways, etc.
- Cost-effective

Outcomes: General Criteria

244

- Experiences no harm, or no injury.
- Doesn't display physical agitation to self or others.
- Eats well balanced meals and gets adequate rest and sleep.
- Interacts appropriately.
- Maintains reality orientation.
- Discusses losses with staff and family/significant others.
- Sets realistic goals for self.

- Identifies aspects of self control over life situation.
- Can concentrate; make decisions.
- Able to relate to others appropriately.
- Has not harmed self or others.
- Demonstrates ability to trust others.
- Uses appropriate communication.
- Performs self-care.
- Maintains anxiety at manageable level.

© 2014 American Nurses Credentialing Center

Planning Improved Outcomes for Pain Management

245

- The patient will:
  - Participate in developing an individualized care plan based on multi-modal therapies to achieve pain relief.
  - Use the Wong-Baker FACES scale (those age 3+, or with developmental or language deficits) to communicate pain.
  - Report pain at an acceptable level.
  - Maintain a daily log of pain, interventions, and responses.
  - Participate in pain management in preparation for discharge.

© 2014 American Nurses Credentialing Center

Planning Improved Outcomes for Anxiety Disorders

246

- The patient will:
  - Recognize signs of anxiety and utilize anxiety reduction skills
  - Verbalize an understanding of the relationship between anxiety and maladaptive coping
  - Deal with stress via coping strategies
    - Thought stopping
    - Relaxation techniques
    - Physical exercise
  - Attend to school/work.

© 2014 American Nurses Credentialing Center

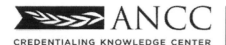
Planning Improved Outcomes for Substance Use Withdrawal

247

- CIWA-Ar, revised: Clinical Institute Withdrawal Assessment for Alcohol: Evidence based tool.
  - Nurse-administered valid and reliable tool to monitor withdrawal and guide medication treatment while hospitalized.
  - 10 distinct symptom areas each scored between 0 to 7.
    - Nausea and vomiting, agitation, tremor, paroxysmal sweats, anxiety, headache/fullness in head, tactile disturbances, auditory disturbances, visual disturbances, orientation, and clouding of sensorium.
  - Score 10 or more: Plan to administer tapered benzodiazepine withdrawal prevention protocol.
- CIWA-B for benzodiazepine withdrawal also available.

© 2014 American Nurses Credentialing Center

Planning Improved Outcomes for Substance Uses

248

- The patient has not experienced injury.
- The patient demonstrates good judgment.
- The patient acknowledges problems and personal responsibility.
- The patient learns adaptive coping mechanism when stressed.
- The patient will engage in patient/family education.
- The patient eats well balanced meals.
- The patient obtains adequate rest.
- The patient is willing to follow through on treatment plan.

© 2014 American Nurses Credentialing Center

Planning Improved Outcomes for Children and Adolescents

249

- Teach proactive interventions systematically.
- Respond warmly to positive behaviors.
- Ignore negative behavior when appropriate.
- Refrain from giving unnecessary commands (demonstrating control when unnecessary).
- Avoid unrealistic demands.
- Use therapeutic play (with children).
- Involve family, school, and other supports.
- Believe reports of bullying, reports of sexual abuse.

© 2014 American Nurses Credentialing Center

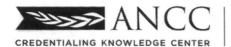

Planning Improved Outcomes for Children and Adolescents: Tools

250

- Therapeutic play
- Pharmacotherapy
- Expressive therapies
- Bibliotherapy
- Children's games
- Storytelling
- Cognitive Behavioral Therapy
- Milieu management

- Special-education
- Computer-based treatment
- Speech and language therapies
- Social skills training
- Sensory integration training
- Music therapy

© 2014 American Nurses Credentialing Center

Planning Improved Outcomes for Autism Spectrum Disorders

251

The patient will:
- Maintain safety (self and others)
- Use socially appropriate behaviors
- Use coping skills
- Gain restorative sleep.

© 2014 American Nurses Credentialing Center

Planning Improved Outcomes for ADHD: Tool

252

- Target Symptoms
  - Problems with social skills
  - Problem-solving
  - School performance
  - Behavioral inhibition
  - Communication
- IOWA Conners Rating Scale
  - Used to substantiate diagnosis of Attention-Deficit Hyperactivity Disorder (ADHD)
  - 3 distinct groups involved in evaluation
    - Parent, teacher, clinician ratings

© 2014 American Nurses Credentialing Center

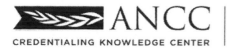
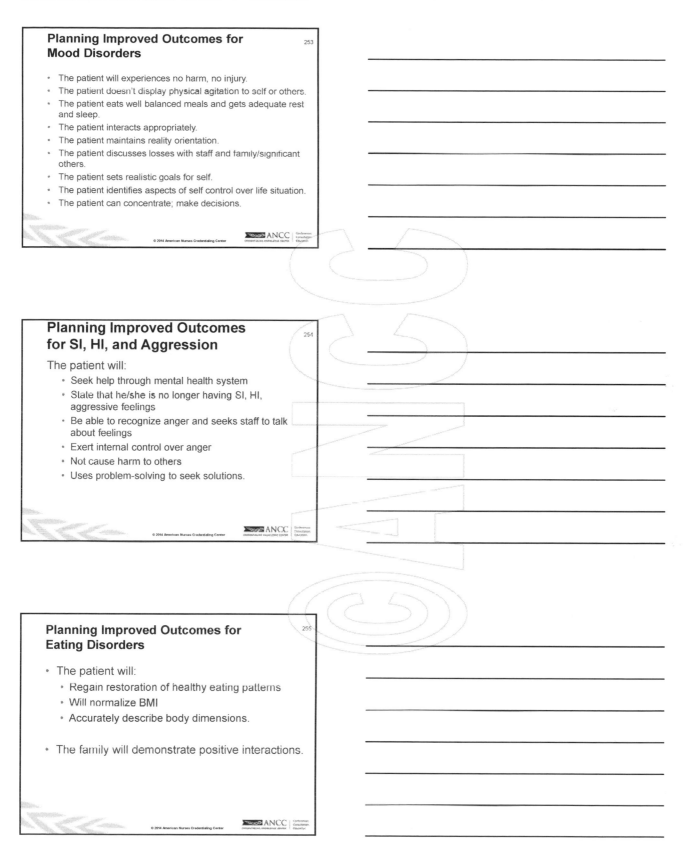

Planning Improved Outcomes for Mood Disorders

253

- The patient will experiences no harm, no injury.
- The patient doesn't display physical agitation to self or others.
- The patient eats well balanced meals and gets adequate rest and sleep.
- The patient interacts appropriately.
- The patient maintains reality orientation.
- The patient discusses losses with staff and family/significant others.
- The patient sets realistic goals for self.
- The patient identifies aspects of self control over life situation.
- The patient can concentrate; make decisions.

© 2014 American Nurses Credentialing Center

Planning Improved Outcomes for SI, HI, and Aggression

254

The patient will:

- Seek help through mental health system
- State that he/she is no longer having SI, HI, aggressive feelings
- Be able to recognize anger and seeks staff to talk about feelings
- Exert internal control over anger
- Not cause harm to others
- Uses problem-solving to seek solutions.

© 2014 American Nurses Credentialing Center

Planning Improved Outcomes for Eating Disorders

255

- The patient will:
  - Regain restoration of healthy eating patterns
  - Will normalize BMI
  - Accurately describe body dimensions.

- The family will demonstrate positive interactions.

© 2014 American Nurses Credentialing Center

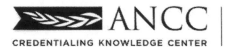
**Planning Improved Outcomes
for Cognitive Disorders**

256

- The patient will achieve optimal functioning across health systems/domains.
- Domains
  - Health perception/health management, value-belief patterns
  - Nutritional-metabolic, elimination patterns
  - Activity-exercise, sleep-rest patterns
  - Cognitive-perceptual patterns
  - Self-perception/self-concept patterns
  - Role-relationship, sexuality-reproductive patterns
  - Coping-stress-tolerance patterns

© 2014 American Nurses Credentialing Center

**CATEGORY II. IMPLEMENTATION
AND EVALUATION**

© 2014 American Nurses Credentialing Center

**CATEGORY II A AND B:
IMPLEMENTATIONS AND
EVALUATIONS**

© 2014 American Nurses Credentialing Center

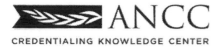
004 : Pharmacological, Biological, & Integrative Therapies (Part 1)

ANCC

004: Learning Objectives 260

1. Discuss nurse-initiated and collaborative strategies related to the administration of psychotropic medications for improved patient outcomes.
2. Discuss the considerations for medication management of the psychiatric mental health population across the life span.

© 2014 American Nurses Credentialing Center ANCC

Implementation: Practice Standard 5 261

- Professional RN carries out both independent and collaborative actions (interventions) that support patient achievement of identified goals and outcomes. Actions aimed at maintaining, facilitating, enhancing, increasing, decreasing, improving patient problems.
  - 5A: Coordination of Care
  - 5B: Health Teaching and Health Promotion
- Examples:
  - Administering psychopharmaceuticals
  - Assessing thought content
  - Engaging psychoeducational groups
  - Enhancing family relationships.

© 2014 American Nurses Credentialing Center ANCC

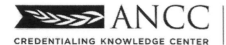
Implementation
262

- Types of Implementations
  - Nurse-initiated
  - Physician initiated
  - Collaborative: Mutual between patient, family, and team.
- Evidence-based implementations incorporate
  - Safety: Crisis management risk management
  - Lifestyle Modification and Psychosocial Functioning: Cognitive/behavioral therapy, education, communication enhancement, coping skills, medication, health promotion, family counseling, and education
  - Health System Effectiveness: Cost containment, fraud, waste, abuse elimination
  - Community and Public Health Implementations: Community health promotion

© 2014 American Nurses Credentialing Center

Pharmacotherapy: Practice Standard 5D
263

- Professional RN incorporates knowledge of pharmacological, biological, and complementary interventions with applied clinical skills to restore the patient's health and prevent disability:
  - Implements the care plan
  - Documents implementations and any modifications, including changes or omissions of the identified plan
  - Provides health teaching and methods for administration and management of medication side effects
  - Documents the patient's understanding of target symptoms, benefits, risks, and alternatives
  - Monitors and documents response and side effects
  - Participates in medication reconciliation.

© 2014 American Nurses Credentialing Center

Pharmacology:
What Drugs Do and How They Do It
264

- Pharmacokinetics: What the body does to the drug.
  - Absorption
  - Metabolism
  - Distribution
  - Elimination
- Pharmacodynamics: What a drug does to the body at specific targeted sites.
  - Receptors
  - Ion channels
  - Enzymes
  - Carrier proteins (re-uptake pumps)

© 2014 American Nurses Credentialing Center

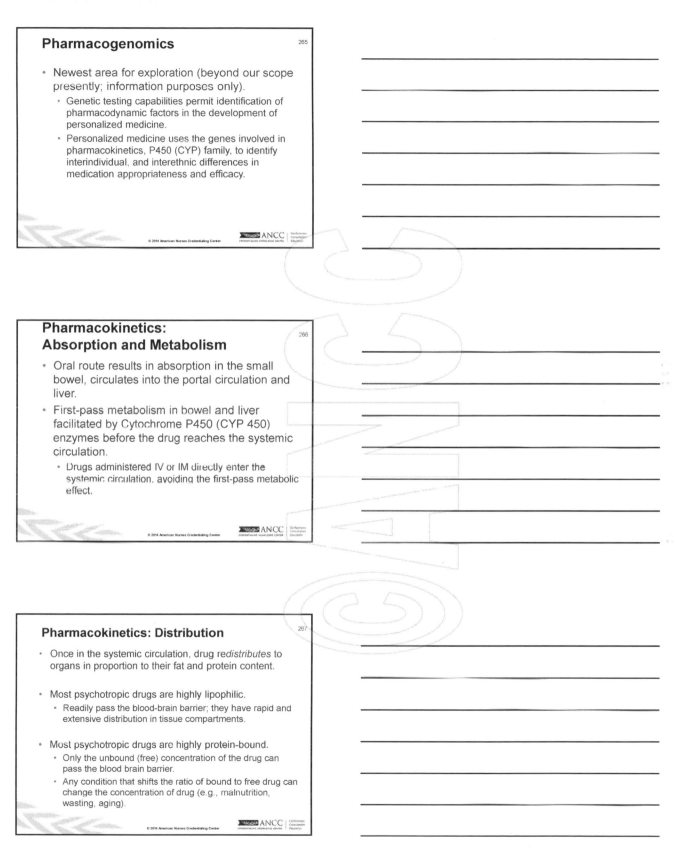

Pharmacogenomics

265

- Newest area for exploration (beyond our scope presently; information purposes only).
  - Genetic testing capabilities permit identification of pharmacodynamic factors in the development of personalized medicine.
  - Personalized medicine uses the genes involved in pharmacokinetics, P450 (CYP) family, to identify interindividual, and interethnic differences in medication appropriateness and efficacy.

Pharmacokinetics: Absorption and Metabolism

266

- Oral route results in absorption in the small bowel, circulates into the portal circulation and liver.
- First-pass metabolism in bowel and liver facilitated by Cytochrome P450 (CYP 450) enzymes before the drug reaches the systemic circulation.
  - Drugs administered IV or IM directly enter the systemic circulation, avoiding the first-pass metabolic effect.

Pharmacokinetics: Distribution

267

- Once in the systemic circulation, drug re*distributes* to organs in proportion to their fat and protein content.

- Most psychotropic drugs are highly lipophilic.
  - Readily pass the blood-brain barrier; they have rapid and extensive distribution in tissue compartments.

- Most psychotropic drugs are highly protein-bound.
  - Only the unbound (free) concentration of the drug can pass the blood brain barrier.
  - Any condition that shifts the ratio of bound to free drug can change the concentration of drug (e.g., malnutrition, wasting, aging).

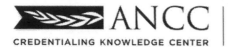
Pharmacokinetics: Elimination

268

- Half-life (T ½): time needed to eliminate (clear) 50% of drug from the plasma.
  - Length of time necessary for drug to reach steady state.
  - Determines how frequently drugs must be taken to maintain desired effect.

- Steady state: Reached when the amount administered per unit time equals the amount eliminated per unit time.
  - Takes five half-lives (T ½) for concentration to build to steady state.
  - Takes five half-lives (T ½) to wash out a drug.

© 2014 American Nurses Credentialing Center

Alterations in Pharmacokinetics

269

- Hepatic CYP450 enzyme interactions can induce or inhibit the metabolism of certain drugs changing the desired concentration levels.
  - Hepatic disease affects liver enzyme activity and first pass metabolism. If a drug has high first pass effects, hepatic disease can result in toxic plasma drug levels.
  - Renal disease or drugs that reduce renal clearance (e.g., NSAIDs) may increase serum concentration of drugs that are excreted by the kidneys (e.g., Lithium).
- If a highly protein bound drug is displaced off its protein, this can result in increased circulating levels of free drug.
- Elders are more sensitive to psychotropics due to decreased intracellular water, protein binding, tissue mass, and increased body fat.

© 2014 American Nurses Credentialing Center

Pharmacodynamics: Receptors

270

- Agonists stimulate biological activity of the receptor.
- Antagonists block or inhibit the actions of agonists, partial agonists, and partial inverse agonists.
- Adverse effects on neurotransmitter receptors that are associated with psychotherapeutic drugs.
  - Anticholinergic: Blockage of muscarinic acetylcholine receptors.
  - Extrapyramidal side effects (EPS): Blockage of dopamine receptors.
  - Sedation: Blockage of histamine receptors.
  - Orthostatic Hypotension: Blockage of adrenergic receptors.
  - Sexual dysfunction, anxiety, akathisia, insomnia, GI upset and diarrhea: Excessive activation of serotonergic receptors.

© 2014 American Nurses Credentialing Center

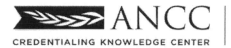
Pharmacodynamics: Ion Channels

271

- Ion channels exist for many ions, including sodium, potassium, chloride, and calcium.

- Neurotransmitters or drugs may be excitatory or inhibitory effects.

Pharmacodynamics: Enzymes

272

- Enzymes are important for drug metabolism.

- Example:
  - Antidepressant drugs that block monoamine oxidases (i.e., MAOIs) decrease the metabolism of catecholamines (i.e., fight or flight hormones), and thus increase the availability of neurotransmitter in the synapse.

Pharmacodynamics: Carrier Proteins

273

- Active transport pumps carry neurotransmitter molecules out of the synapse and back into the presynaptic neuron.

- When reuptake pumps are blocked (inhibited), the concentration of certain neurotransmitters or ions build up in the synapse (extracellular space between neurons).
  - Example:
    - SSRIs block re-uptake of serotonin, increasing availability in the synapse.

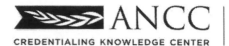

Conferences.
Consultation.
Education.

Pharmacology Terminology

274

- Potency: The relative dose required to achieve certain effects.
  - Haldol (5mg) is more potent than Thorazine (100mg) less is needed to achieve the same therapeutic effect.

- Therapeutic Index: A relative measure of the toxicity or safety of a drug defined as the ratio of the median toxic dose to the median effective dose.
  - The therapeutic index of Lithium is quite low and requires careful monitoring of serum levels.

- Tolerance: The process of becoming less responsive to a particular drug as it is administered over time.

Broad Classes of Psychotropic Drugs

275

- Antipsychotics/neuroleptics/major tranquilizers: Psychosis
- Antidepressants: Depression, pain
- Antimanic/mood stabilizers/anticonvulsants: Bipolar
- Antianxiety/anxiolytics/minor tranquilizers: Anxiety
- Psychostimulants: Attention deficit hyperactivity disorder
- Cognitive enhancers: Dementia
  - Generally, symptom management is the treatment target. Additionally, symptoms may cut across the drug/illness classes.
    - Example: Drugs from one class (i.e., antidepressants) can treat disorders (i.e., anxiety) assigned to another class.

Implementations: Psychotic Disorders

276

- Trust building
- Patient/family education
  - Illness symptoms or progressions
  - Illness management
  - Support services
- Case management
- Milieu therapy
- Group therapy (Reality Oriented)
- Psychopharmacology

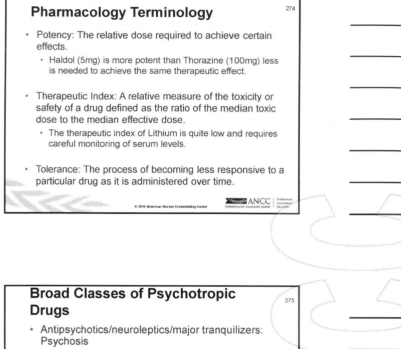

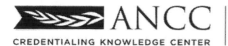

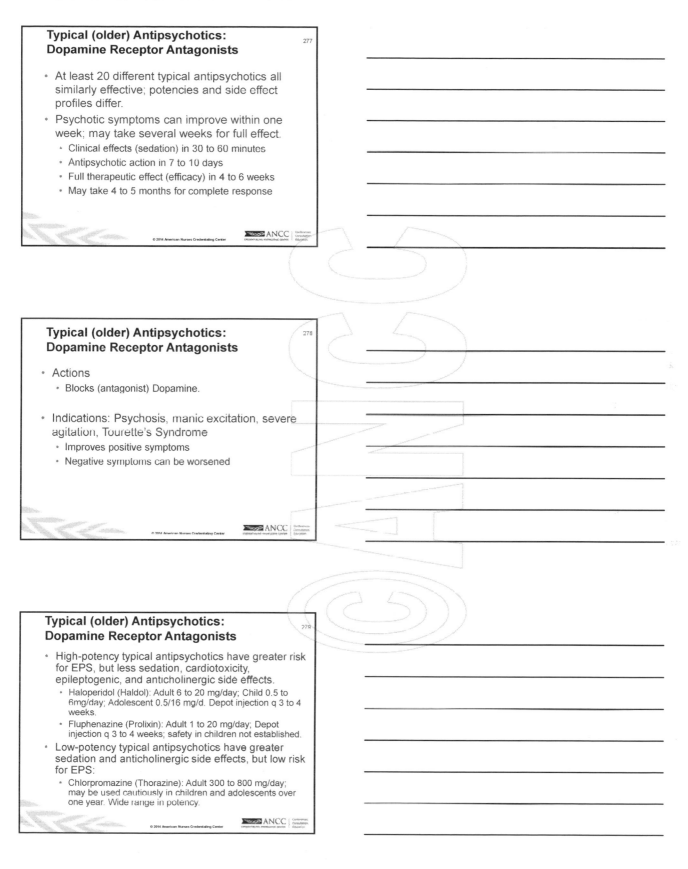

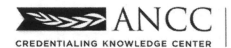

ANCC | Conferences. Consultation. Education.

CREDENTIALING KNOWLEDGE CENTER

Atypical (newer) Antipsychotics: Nursing Care Planning Strategies

280

- Baseline measures: Weight, waist circumference, BP, fasting plasma glucose, fasting lipid profile. Assess family history of obesity, dyslipidemia, hypertension, or cardiovascular disease.
- Concerns
  - Weight gain: Monitor weight and BMI (foster exercise, nutrition).
  - Sedation: May be best to administer at bedtime.
  - Hyperglycemia/ketoacidosis: Monitor fasting plasma glucose.
  - Agranulocytosis: Monitor for flu-like symptoms, sore throat, signs of infection). Problem if white blood cell count falls below 2,000/mm3.
  - EPS: Administer anticholinergics to reduce motor symptoms.
- Advocate medication change to another atypical antipsychotic for overweight, obese, pre-diabetic/diabetic, hypertensive, or dyslipidemic patients.

© 2014 American Nurses Credentialing Center

Atypical (newer) Antipsychotics:

clozapine (Clozaril, Leponex)

281

- Not a first-line treatment due to life threatening side effects:
  - Agranulocytosis: Monitor WBC with differential counts weekly.
  - Seizures: May increase related to dose.
  - Hyperglycemia with ketoacidosis: Monitor fasting plasma glucose.
  - Dyslipidemia: Monitor lipids (amount of fat in blood), weight
  - Pulmonary embolism.
  - Myocarditis: Monitor ECG.
  - Neuroleptic Malignant Syndrome (NMS): Monitor temperature, mental status. Potentially fatal!
- Usual dosage range: 300 to 450 mg/day.

© 2014 American Nurses Credentialing Center

Atypical (newer) Antipsychotics: Dosage Ranges

282

- Risperidone (Risperdal)
  - Adult: 2 to 8mg/day
  - Child/elders: .5 to 2 mg/day
  - Long-acting (Consta): 25 to 50mg depot IM q two weeks
  - Risks: EPS and hyperprolactinemia at dosages greater than 6mg/day
- Olanzapine (Zyprexa)
  - Adult: 10 to 20mg/day
  - Child (not officially recommended, but used at 2.5 to 10 mg/day)
  - Significant weight gain
- Zyprexa Relprevv (long acting)
  - Administered every 2 to 4 weeks

- Quetiapine (Seroquel)
  - Adult: 150 to 750 mg/day
  - Child: (not officially recommended, but used at 25 to 500 mg/day)
  - Sedation and weight gain can be problematic
- Ziprasidone (Geodon)
  - Adult: 40 to 200mg/day
  - Child: (not officially recommended)
  - May have activating effects at low doses. Risk of QTC prolongation – monitor ECG. Weight gain is uncommon.
  - Take with 500 calorie meal.

© 2014 American Nurses Credentialing Center

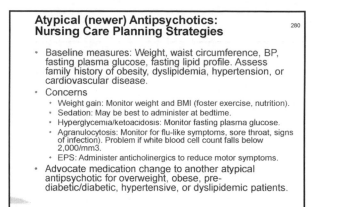

© 2014 American Nurses Credentialing Center

94

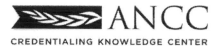
Atypical (newer) Antipsychotics: Dosage Ranges
283

- Aripiprazole (Abilify)
  - Adult: 10 to 15mg/ bid
  - Child: 2 to 15 mg/day
  - Extended Release: Abilify Maintena: 200-400 mg IM monthly depot
  - Risks: Akathisia, agitation, insomnia, headache, weight gain
- Paliperidone (Invega)
  - Adult: 6 to 12mg/day
  - Child: Safety and efficacy not established
  - Risks: Akathisia and hyperprolactinemia
- Asenapine (Saphris)
  - Adult: 5 to 10 mg SL
  - Child: Safety and efficacy not established
  - Risks: Somnolence, oral hypoesthesia, anaphylaxis

- Iloperidone (Fanapt)
  - Adult: 6 to 12 mg bid
  - Child: Safety and efficacy not established
  - Risks: Dizziness, somnolence, orthostatic hypotension
- Lurasidone (Latuda)
  - Adult: 40 to 80mg/day (take with at least 350 calories)
  - Child: Safety and efficacy not established
  - Risks: Somnolence, akathisia, nausea, parkinsonism

© 2014 American Nurses Credentialing Center

Assessment: Abnormal Involuntary Movements (AIMS)
284

- Movement disorder assessment : A critical role for the professional RN
  - Regular ratings pre and post neuroleptic administration (in particular) and also with other psychotropics help detect whether medication vs. medical-illness induced changes in motor response and fluidity.
  - Presence and severity of each type of abnormal movement or rigidity is rated none to severe.
    - Sitting, standing, or walking
    - Tongue, mouth movements
    - Rapid finger-thumb tapping
    - Passively flex and extend arms for cogwheel rigidity

© 2014 American Nurses Credentialing Center

Neurological Adverse Side Effects of Antipsychotics
205

- Extrapyramidal symptoms (EPS) are abnormal, involuntary movements
  - Akathisia: Subjective feeling of muscular discomfort and restlessness
  - Dystonia: Slow, sustained muscle contractions or spasms, can result in oculogyric crisis, blepharospasm, or glossopharyngeal dystonias
  - Parkinsonism: Muscle stiffness, cogwheel rigidity, shuffling gait, stooped posture, drooling, or slow resting tremor
  - Tardive Dyskinesia (TD): Perioral (around the mouth and tongue) abnormal movements, tongue, and lip smacking

© 2014 American Nurses Credentialing Center

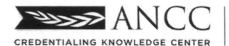
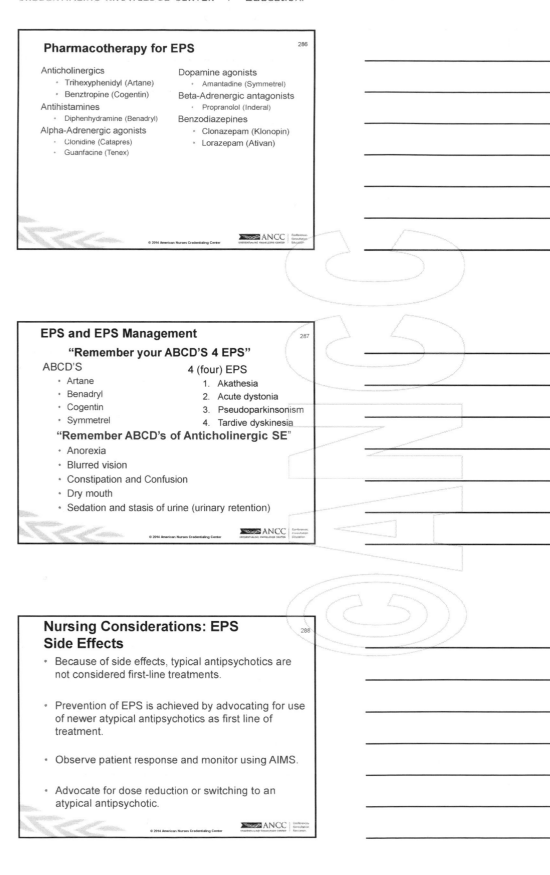

Pharmacotherapy for EPS 286

Anticholinergics
- Trihexyphenidyl (Artane)
- Benztropine (Cogentin)

Antihistamines
- Diphenhydramine (Benadryl)

Alpha-Adrenergic agonists
- Clonidine (Catapres)
- Guanfacine (Tenex)

Dopamine agonists
- Amantadine (Symmetrel)

Beta-Adrenergic antagonists
- Propranolol (Inderal)

Benzodiazepines
- Clonazepam (Klonopin)
- Lorazepam (Ativan)

© 2014 American Nurses Credentialing Center

EPS and EPS Management 287

"Remember your ABCD'S 4 EPS"

ABCD'S
- Artane
- Benadryl
- Cogentin
- Symmetrel

4 (four) EPS
1. Akathesia
2. Acute dystonia
3. Pseudoparkinsonism
4. Tardive dyskinesia

"Remember ABCD's of Anticholinergic SE"
- Anorexia
- Blurred vision
- Constipation and Confusion
- Dry mouth
- Sedation and stasis of urine (urinary retention)

© 2014 American Nurses Credentialing Center

Nursing Considerations: EPS Side Effects 288

- Because of side effects, typical antipsychotics are not considered first-line treatments.

- Prevention of EPS is achieved by advocating for use of newer atypical antipsychotics as first line of treatment.

- Observe patient response and monitor using AIMS.

- Advocate for dose reduction or switching to an atypical antipsychotic.

© 2014 American Nurses Credentialing Center

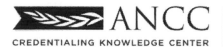
Non-Neurological Effects of Typical Antipsychotics and Treatment Strategies

289

- Anticholinergic Symptoms
  - Dry mouth and nose: Rinse mouth with water, saline spray for nasal congestion, sugar-free candy, and increased hydration,
  - Blurred vision: Pilocarpine eye drops (for short-term use), reassurance that blurred vision will improve, caution to not perform any dangerous tasks until blurred vision remits,
  - Urinary retention: Bethanechol (Urecholine), and
  - Constipation: Laxative, ambulation.
- Anticholinergic Toxicity
  - Agitation, disorientation to time, person, and place; hallucinations; seizures; high fever; dilated pupils. Stupor and coma may ensue; elders are especially vulnerable. "Dry as a bone, red as a beet, hot as a hare, blind as a bat, and mad as a hatter," and
  - Treatment: Discontinue the causative agents, observe closely for safety, and administer medication to reverse symptoms.

© 2014 American Nurses Credentialing Center

Non-Neurological Effects of Typical Antipsychotics and Treatment Strategies

290

- Sedation
  - Consider risk for falls, orthostatic hypotension, warnings about driving and operating equipment; consider bedtime dosing, lower dose or switch drugs.
- Orthostatic Hypotension
  - Measure BP before and after first dose; measure sitting, lying, standing; teach patient to rise slowly.
- GI Discomfort
  - If no contraindications, take medication with meals.
- Weight Gain
  - Teach about increased risks, promote exercise and healthy diet.
  - Increased Prolactin levels lead to breast enlargement, Galactorrhea, and sexual dysfunction, especially troublesome for adolescent males (adverse effect should be thoroughly discussed before treatment begins).
- Photosensitivity
  - Wear sunscreen and wide brim hats when outdoors.

© 2014 American Nurses Credentialing Center

Neuroleptic Malignant Syndrome (NMS) Associated With Antipsychotics

291

- Life-threatening complication associated with antipsychotic (neuroleptic) therapy; can occur anytime in treatment.
  - Motor and behavioral symptoms include: muscular rigidity, dystonia, akinesia, mutism, obtundation, agitation.
  - Autonomic symptoms include: hyperpyrexia, sweating, increased pulse, and BP.
- Treatment: Immediate discontinuation of medication; medical support to cool the patient; monitor vital signs, electrolytes, fluid balance, renal output; treatment of elevated temperature.

© 2014 American Nurses Credentialing Center

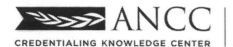
Antipsychotic Indications in Children and Adolescents

292

- Psychoses, agitated self-injurious behaviors that may accompany Developmental Disabilities, Neurodevelopmental Disorders, Conduct Disorder, and Tourette's Syndrome.
  - Work fast and are more robust than Lithium.
- First-episode patients should remain on antipsychotic treatment for one to two years to prevent relapses.
  - Adverse effects are similar to adults.

© 2014 American Nurses Credentialing Center

Implementations: Mood Disorders

293

- Protect from self-harm or injury due to hyperactivity
- Protect from harm from others
- Monitor responses to medications when beginning effectiveness
- Help restore nutritional status and adequate sleep/rest
- Help improve interactions
- Patient/family education
- Enhance self-esteem, hygiene
- Help taking control over life
- Help in confronting anger turned inward or outward

© 2014 American Nurses Credentialing Center

Depression: Monoamine Hypothesis (Theory)

294

- Deficits in the monoamine neurotransmitter system (effects serotonin, norepinephrine, dopamine) causes depression.

- Evidence: All antidepressants increase one or more of the monoamines.

© 2014 American Nurses Credentialing Center

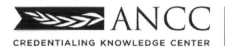
Classes of Antidepressants

295

- Tricyclic antidepressants (TCAs)
- Monoamine oxidase inhibitors (MAOIs)
- Selective serotonin reuptake inhibitors (SSRIs)
- Dual serotonin and norepinephrine reuptake inhibitors (SNRIs)
- Norepinephrine dopamine reuptake inhibitors (NDRIs)
- Serotonin 2 antagonist/reuptake inhibitors (SARIs)
- Alpha 2 Antagonist/Noradrenaline and Specific Serotonergic Agent (NaSSAs)

© 2014 American Nurses Credentialing Center

TCAs and Usual Adult Daily Dosage Ranges

296

- Imipramine (Tofranil): 150 to 300mg
- Desipramine (Norpramin): 150 to 300mg
- Trimipramine (Surmontil): 150 to 300mg
- Amitriptyline (Elavil, Endep): 150 to 300mg
- Nortriptyline (Pamelor, Aventyl): 5 to 150mg
- Protriptyline (Vivactil): 15 to 60mg
- Amoxapine (Asendin): 150 to 400mg
- Doxepin (Adapin, Sinequan): 150 to 300mg
- Maprotiline (Ludiomil): 150 to 230mg
- Clomipramine (Anafranil): 130 to 250 mg (adult); 50 to 200 mg (children/adol)

© 2014 American Nurses Credentialing Center

TCAs Indications

297

- Depression
- Obsessive-compulsive disorder
  - Clomipramine (Anafranil)
- Chronic pain
  - Neurogenic pain, trigeminal neuralgia, diabetic neuropathy, sciatica, and fibromyalgia
- Sleep disorders
  - Insomnia or cataplexy

© 2014 American Nurses Credentialing Center

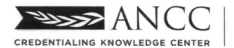
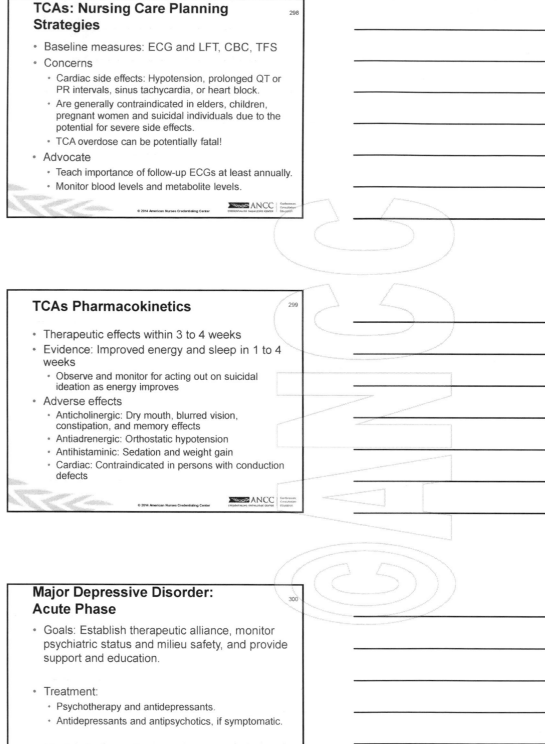

TCAs: Nursing Care Planning Strategies

298

- Baseline measures: ECG and LFT, CBC, TFS
- Concerns
  - Cardiac side effects: Hypotension, prolonged QT or PR intervals, sinus tachycardia, or heart block.
  - Are generally contraindicated in elders, children, pregnant women and suicidal individuals due to the potential for severe side effects.
  - TCA overdose can be potentially fatal!
- Advocate
  - Teach importance of follow-up ECGs at least annually.
  - Monitor blood levels and metabolite levels.

© 2014 American Nurses Credentialing Center

TCAs Pharmacokinetics

299

- Therapeutic effects within 3 to 4 weeks
- Evidence: Improved energy and sleep in 1 to 4 weeks
  - Observe and monitor for acting out on suicidal ideation as energy improves
- Adverse effects
  - Anticholinergic: Dry mouth, blurred vision, constipation, and memory effects
  - Antiadrenergic: Orthostatic hypotension
  - Antihistaminic: Sedation and weight gain
  - Cardiac: Contraindicated in persons with conduction defects

© 2014 American Nurses Credentialing Center

Major Depressive Disorder: Acute Phase

300

- Goals: Establish therapeutic alliance, monitor psychiatric status and milieu safety, and provide support and education.

- Treatment:
  - Psychotherapy and antidepressants.
  - Antidepressants and antipsychotics, if symptomatic.

- Monitor for side effects and increase in SI: Re-assess adequacy of response in 4 to 8 weeks.

© 2014 American Nurses Credentialing Center

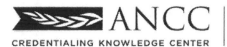
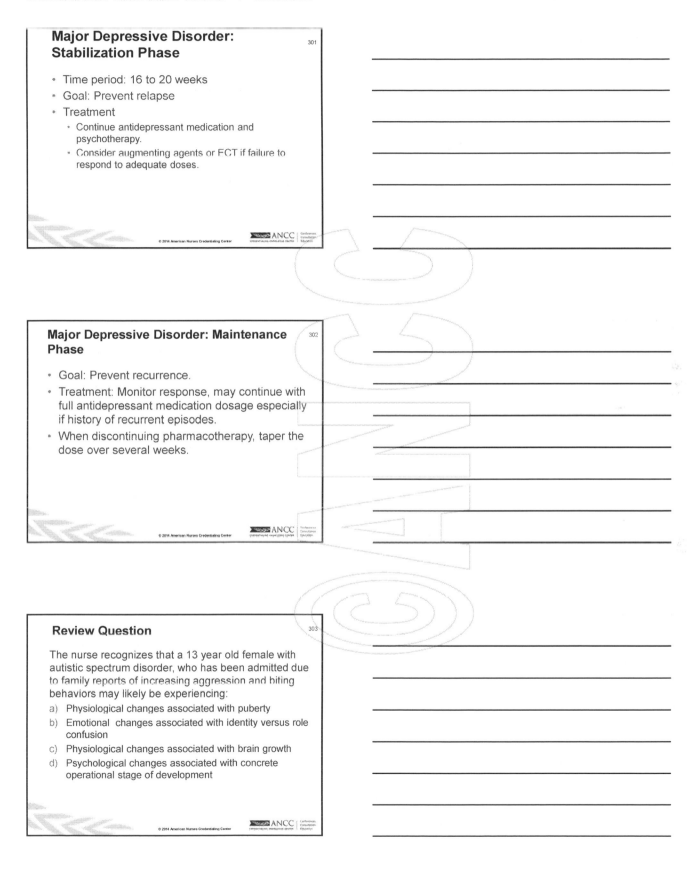

Major Depressive Disorder: Stabilization Phase

301

- Time period: 16 to 20 weeks
- Goal: Prevent relapse
- Treatment
  - Continue antidepressant medication and psychotherapy.
  - Consider augmenting agents or ECT if failure to respond to adequate doses.

© 2014 American Nurses Credentialing Center

Major Depressive Disorder: Maintenance Phase

302

- Goal: Prevent recurrence.
- Treatment: Monitor response, may continue with full antidepressant medication dosage especially if history of recurrent episodes.
- When discontinuing pharmacotherapy, taper the dose over several weeks.

© 2014 American Nurses Credentialing Center

Review Question

303

The nurse recognizes that a 13 year old female with autistic spectrum disorder, who has been admitted due to family reports of increasing aggression and biting behaviors may likely be experiencing:

a) Physiological changes associated with puberty
b) Emotional changes associated with identity versus role confusion
c) Physiological changes associated with brain growth
d) Psychological changes associated with concrete operational stage of development

© 2014 American Nurses Credentialing Center

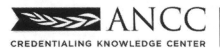

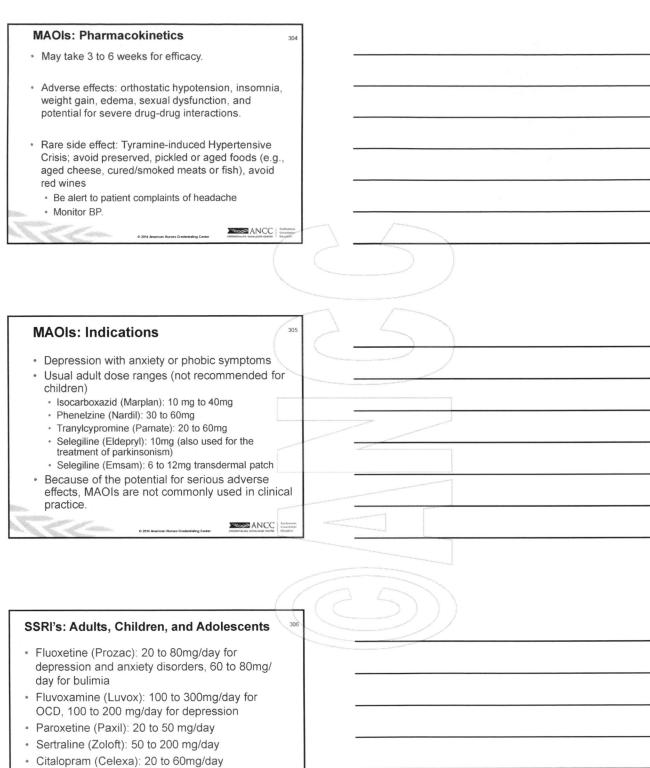

MAOIs: Pharmacokinetics

304

- May take 3 to 6 weeks for efficacy.

- Adverse effects: orthostatic hypotension, insomnia, weight gain, edema, sexual dysfunction, and potential for severe drug-drug interactions.

- Rare side effect: Tyramine-induced Hypertensive Crisis; avoid preserved, pickled or aged foods (e.g., aged cheese, cured/smoked meats or fish), avoid red wines
  - Be alert to patient complaints of headache
  - Monitor BP.

© 2014 American Nurses Credentialing Center

MAOIs: Indications

305

- Depression with anxiety or phobic symptoms
- Usual adult dose ranges (not recommended for children)
  - Isocarboxazid (Marplan): 10 mg to 40mg
  - Phenelzine (Nardil): 30 to 60mg
  - Tranylcypromine (Parnate): 20 to 60mg
  - Selegiline (Eldepryl): 10mg (also used for the treatment of parkinsonism)
  - Selegiline (Emsam): 6 to 12mg transdermal patch
- Because of the potential for serious adverse effects, MAOIs are not commonly used in clinical practice.

© 2014 American Nurses Credentialing Center

SSRI's: Adults, Children, and Adolescents

306

- Fluoxetine (Prozac): 20 to 80mg/day for depression and anxiety disorders, 60 to 80mg/day for bulimia
- Fluvoxamine (Luvox): 100 to 300mg/day for OCD, 100 to 200 mg/day for depression
- Paroxetine (Paxil): 20 to 50 mg/day
- Sertraline (Zoloft): 50 to 200 mg/day
- Citalopram (Celexa): 20 to 60mg/day
- Escitalopram (Lexapro): 10 to 20mg/day
- vilazodone (Viibryd): 10 to 40mg/day

© 2014 American Nurses Credentialing Center

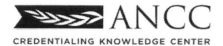
SSRI Indications

307

* Depression, OCD, panic disorder, social anxiety disorder, PTSD, eating disorders, and borderline personality disorder.
* Pharmacokinetics: Therapeutic effects may take 3 to 6 weeks for depression and 12 to 16 weeks for OCD.
    * Observe for activation of known or unknown bipolar disorder and/or suicidal ideation (Black Box Warning).
    * Inform parents or guardian of this risk so they can help observe child or adolescent patterns.
* Adolescents often receive adult dose, but doses are slightly less for children.

SSRIs: Adverse Effects

308

* Common: anxiety, agitation, akathisia, insomnia, nausea, diarrhea, sexual dysfunction (bupropion (Wellbutrin) treats sexual dysfunction or switch to another medication).
* Serotonin Syndrome: diarrhea, restlessness, extreme agitation, hyper-reflexia and autonomic instability, myoclonus, seizures, hyperthermia, rigidity, delirium, coma, possible death. Serotonin Syndrome causes "HARM" (Hyperthermia, Autonomic instability, Rigidity, Myoclonus) .
* Serotonin Discontinuation Syndrome: agitation, nausea, dysequilibrium, and dysphoria; tapering off medication is advised.

SARIs and SNRIs: Novel Antidepressant Agents

309

* Serotonin-2 Antagonist Reuptake Inhibitors (SARIs)
    * Nefazodone (Serzone): 300 to 600mg/day
        * Risk of hepatotoxicity, so not a first-line medication
    * trazodone (Desyrel): 150 to 600mg/day (Oleptro – SR formulation)
        * Generally used for insomnia due to sedative properties
        * Risk for priapism in males
        * Caution with children and adolescents

* Serotonin/Norepinephrine Reuptake Inhibitors (SNRIs)
    * Venlafaxine (Effexor): 75 to 225 mg/day. Extended release available
    * Desvenlafaxine (Pristiq): 50 to 100 mg/day adults; safety/efficacy not established in children
    * Duloxetine (Cymbalta): 40 to 60mg/day

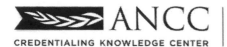
NDRIs, NASSAs, and Ketamine: Novel Antidepressant Agents
310

- Norepinephrine/Dopamine Reuptake Inhibitor (NDRIs)
  - Bupropion (Wellbutrin; Zyban): 225 to 450mg/day
    - Also SR and XL forms
    - May increase seizure risk: Avoid if hx of seizures or bulimia
    - Commonly used as an augmenting agent with other antidepressants, no sexual side effects, used for smoking cessation
    - Used to treat ADHD in children at 100 to 250 mg/day

- Alpha 2 Antagonist/Noradrenaline and Specific Serotonergic Agent (NaSSA)
  - Mirtazapine (Remeron): 15 to 45mg at bedtime.
    - Antihistamine effects: Highly sedating at lower doses but also causes weight gain

- Ketamine IV – Serial treatment for intractable depression (being tried in some areas)

© 2014 American Nurses Credentialing Center   ANCC

Considerations for Women
311

- Pregnancy
  - Most malformations (teratogenic effects) occur during the 3rd to 8th week of gestation (embryonic period).

- Postpartum
  - High-risk time or onset or relapse of psychiatric illnesses.
  - Consider risk versus benefit of the impact of untreated illness on maternal-infant attachment (bonding).
  - All psychotropics are secreted in breast milk.

- Postmenopausal
  - Estrogen replacement plus SSRI or SNRIs are effective for maintenance and prevention of recurrence.

© 2014 American Nurses Credentialing Center   ANCC

Considerations for Children and Adolescents
312

- Unlike adults, children may not respond to TCAs.

- Children and adolescents do respond well to SSRIs and perhaps to other classes of antidepressants as well.

- FDA Black Box Warning: 2% to 3% greater risk of suicidal behavior in children taking antidepressants.

© 2014 American Nurses Credentialing Center   ANCC

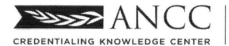
Review Question 313

The FDA's black box warning appended on all antidepressant medication labels indicate:

a) Increased risk of suicide in young adults 18-24 years.

b) Increase risk for Stevens Johnson Syndrome.

c) Increase risk for serotonin syndrome among young adolescents 15-20.

d) Fatalities have occurred if simultaneously taking St. John's wort.

© 2014 American Nurses Credentialing Center

Bipolar Disorder 314

- Theoretical mechanisms:
  - Sensitization: Recurring stressors and episodes can predispose an individual to increased vulnerability to future episodes in a long-lasting fashion.
  - Kindling: Repeated intermittent sub-threshold stimulation of a given region of the brain eventually leads to full-blown amygdala seizures (affective episodes).
- Evidence. Anticonvulsants and Lithium have anti-kindling effects
- Post, 2003. Pediatric bipolar disorder.

© 2014 American Nurses Credentialing Center

Bipolar Disorder:
Acute and Initiation Phases 315

- Goals: Manage symptoms of agitation, aggression, and impulsivity; return to usual levels of psychosocial functioning. If depressed, avoid precipitation of manic episode.
- Treatment:
  - Severe mania or mixed episodes: Lithium or valproate in combination with an antipsychotic.
  - For less severely ill: Monotherapy with lithium, valproate, or an atypical antipsychotic.
  - If symptoms are inadequately controlled after 10 to 14 days, another first-line medication may be added.
- Baseline:
  - Lithium: BUN, creatinine, thyroid, ECG, pregnancy.
  - Valproate: Assess for hepatic, hematological, and bleeding abnormalities and pregnancy.

© 2014 American Nurses Credentialing Center

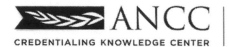
Bipolar Disorder: Stabilization and Maintenance Phases

316

- Goals: Prevent relapse and recurrence, reduce sub-threshold symptoms, reduce suicide risk, reduce cycling frequency or milder degrees of mood instability, and improve overall function.

- Treatment: Maintenance medication is recommended following a manic or depressive episode. Monitor lithium, carbamazepine, or valproate levels, hematologic, and hepatic functioning at least every six months.

© 2014 American Nurses Credentialing Center

Lithium: Management of Bipolar Disorder

317

- Indications: Acute mania and mood stabilization
- Usual adult dosage: 900 to 1,800 mg/day in divided doses:
    - Long half-life yet narrow therapeutic index
    - Response in acute mania may take 7 to 14 days.
- Narrow therapeutic index requires frequent physical exams and labs.
- Therapeutic serum blood level range
    - Acute episode: 0.8 to 1.4 mEq per L
    - Maintenance: 0.4 to 1.0 mEq per L

© 2014 American Nurses Credentialing Center

Lithium: Management of Bipolar Disorder

318

- Check for family history of kidney disease, diabetes, and hypertension.
- Baseline: Before taking any medication that is cleared by the kidneys, renal function should be assessed, and then again every six months, routine lab, and physical exams required.
    - BUN, creatinine clearance (24 hr. urine), 24 hr. urine volume, 12 hr. fluid deprivation test, Glomerular Filtration Rate (GFR).

© 2014 American Nurses Credentialing Center

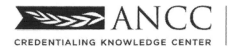

Lithium: Management of Bipolar Disorder

319

- Common adverse effects: Tremor (propranolol [Inderal] and reduced caffeine intake may reduce tremor), weight gain, sedation, and stomach upset (take with meals to reduce GI upset).
- Fluids and Electrolytes: Avoid dehydration, overhydration, and excessive salt.
- Drug-drug interactions:
  - NSAIDS, hydrochlorothiazide, and ACE inhibitors cause lithium levels to be high.
  - Caffeine increases GFR (urinate more) leading to lowered lithium levels.

© 2014 American Nurses Credentialing Center

Lithium: Management of Bipolar Disorder

320

- Lithium toxicity: A medical emergency
  - Signs: Diarrhea, nausea, vomiting, drowsiness, tremor, muscle weakness, giddiness, ataxia, vertical nystagmus, tinnitus, diabetes insipidus, and multiorgan toxicity
  - Hold (have discontinued immediately), emesis, lavage, and dialysis may be required
- Teratogenic potential
  - Lithium is toxic to embryonic development. Use with caution in women of reproductive ages.

© 2011 American Nurses Credentialing Center

Anticonvulsants:
Management of Bipolar Disorder

321

- Valproate/divalproex Depakene/Depakote): 1,200 to 1,500 mg/day (adult); up to 20mg/kg/day (child/adol)
  - Used for acute mania; less effective for maintenance and bipolar depression
  - Therapeutic level: 40-100 mcg/ml
- Carbamazepine (Tegretol): 400 to 1,200 mg/day; up to 20-30 mg/kg/day (child/adol)
  - Second-line augmenting agent for acute mania
  - Risk for agranulocytosis: Monitor WBC q2 wks x 2 mo then q3 mos
  - Therapeutic level: 4-12 mg/L

© 2011 American Nurses Credentialing Center

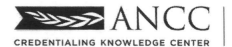
Anticonvulsants:

Management of Bipolar Disorder

322

- Gabapentin (Neurontin): 900 to 1,800 mg/day
  - Well tolerated; questionably effective. Good anti-anxiety and pain control effects
- Lamotrigine (Lamictal): 100 to 200 mg/day
  - Indicated for bipolar maintenance; useful for bipolar depression
  - Risk of rare toxic, potentially fatal necrolysis skin condition (Stevens-Johnson Syndrome). Start very low and go slow; 25mg every other day x 2 weeks
  - Children and adolescents have higher incidence of life-threatening rash than adults
- Topiramate (Topamax): 50 to 300 mg/day
  - Useful adjunct in bipolar disorder; not first-line
  - May actually cause weight loss

© 2014 American Nurses Credentialing Center

Anticonvulsants:

Management of Bipolar Disorder

323

- Therapeutic effects begin after days; mood stabilization may take weeks to months. Never discontinued abruptly.
- Common transient adverse effects:
  - Nausea, diarrhea, or sedation
- Common adverse effects:
  - Weight gain: Monitor weight and BMI, diet and exercise (lamotrigine (Lamictal) and topiramate (Topamax) have lowest risk)
  - Tremor: Consider low dose beta-blocker
  - Increased risk for thrombocytopenia: Monitor prothrombin time, bleeding tendencies
  - Risk for agranulocytosis (i.e., especially with carbamazepine [Tegretol]): monitor WBC with differentials

© 2014 American Nurses Credentialing Center

Antipsychotics:

Management of Bipolar Disorder

324

- Atypical antipsychotics:
  - Asenapine (Saphris), ziprasidone (Geodon),olanzapine (Zyprexa), quetiapine (Seroquel), risperidone (Risperdal), aripiprazole (Abilify) are useful for treatment of acute mania

- Symbyax is FDA approved for bipolar depression.
  - Combination of olanzapine (Zyprexa) and fluoxetine (Prozac)

© 2014 American Nurses Credentialing Center

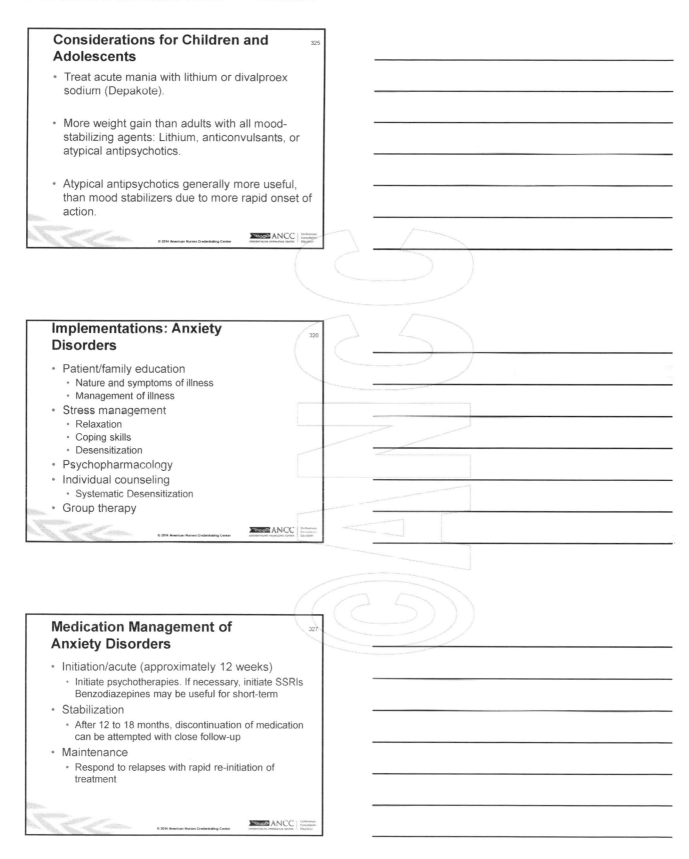

Considerations for Children and Adolescents

325

- Treat acute mania with lithium or divalproex sodium (Depakote).

- More weight gain than adults with all mood-stabilizing agents: Lithium, anticonvulsants, or atypical antipsychotics.

- Atypical antipsychotics generally more useful, than mood stabilizers due to more rapid onset of action.

© 2014 American Nurses Credentialing Center

Implementations: Anxiety Disorders

320

- Patient/family education
  - Nature and symptoms of illness
  - Management of illness
- Stress management
  - Relaxation
  - Coping skills
  - Desensitization
- Psychopharmacology
- Individual counseling
  - Systematic Desensitization
- Group therapy

© 2014 American Nurses Credentialing Center

Medication Management of Anxiety Disorders

327

- Initiation/acute (approximately 12 weeks)
  - Initiate psychotherapies. If necessary, initiate SSRIs Benzodiazepines may be useful for short-term
- Stabilization
  - After 12 to 18 months, discontinuation of medication can be attempted with close follow-up
- Maintenance
  - Respond to relapses with rapid re-initiation of treatment

© 2014 American Nurses Credentialing Center

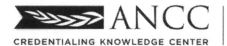

Medication Management of Anxiety

328

- SSRIs are first-line treatments for chronic anxiety symptoms associated with panic disorder, phobias, social anxiety disorder, and OCD.
  - Therapeutic effects may take 2 to 4 weeks.
- Benzodiazepines are used for acute anxiety and agitation.
  - Potentiates the effect of GABA, inhibiting neurotransmission in limbic system and cortex.
  - Anti-anxiety effects in 30 to 60 minutes.
  - Use lowest possible effective dose for shortest possible period of time.
  - Side effects: Drowsiness, fatigue, depression, dizziness, ataxia, slurred speech, weakness, and forgetfulness.

© 2014 American Nurses Credentialing Center

Medication Management of Anxiety: Benzodiazepines

329

- Half-lives: Longer half-lives = Less frequent dosing, less variation in plasma concentration; less severe withdrawal, less rebound.
- Benzodiazepines with long half-lives
  - Diazepam (Valium): 4 to 40 mg/day
- Benzodiazepines with intermediate half-lives
  - Clonazepam (Klonopin): 1 to 6 mg /day (adult), 0.5 to 2.0 mg/d (child)
- Benzodiazepines with short half-lives:
  - Alprazolam (Xanax): 0.5 to 10 mg/day (adult); up to 1.5 mg/day (child)
  - Lorazepam, (Ativan): 1 to 6 mg/day
- Benzodiazepines safe with liver failure
  - "LOT": Lorazepam (Ativan), oxazepam (Serax), temazepam (Restoril).

© 2014 American Nurses Credentialing Center

Medication Management of Anxiety Disorders: Discontinuation

330

- Because of the risk of psychological dependence, long-term use should be carefully monitored. The drugs should be tapered at discontinuation.
- Discontinuation syndromes depend on the length of time on drug, the dosage taken, the rate of taper, and the half-life. The higher the dose, the shorter the half-life, the more severe the withdrawal symptoms.
- Withdrawal symptoms include: Anxiety, nervousness, diaphoresis, restlessness, irritability, fatigue, light-headedness, tremor, insomnia, weakness, risk for seizures, and death.

© 2014 American Nurses Credentialing Center

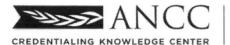
Medication Management of Anxiety

331

- Serotonin Partial-agonist: Buspirone (BuSpar)
  - Usual dose: 20 to 30 mg/day
  - Therapeutic effects may take 4 weeks
  - No physiological dependence
- Antidepressant: Clomipramine (Anafranil)
  - Treats anxiety. OCD
  - Usual dose: 25mg titrated to 100 mg qd
- Beta-blockers: Propranolol (Inderal)
  - Useful for performance anxiety where tremor might be a problem
  - Usual dose: 10 to 20 mg bid or tid

© 2014 American Nurses Credentialing Center

Medication Management of Anxiety in Children and Adolescents

332

- Generally started on a broad-spectrum SSRI
  - If ADHD symptoms also present, a stimulant or bupropion may be added as an adjunct.
  - If insomnia, hyperstartle, or hyperarousal symptoms are problematic, alpha-agonists such as clonidine (Catapres) or guanfacine (Tenex) may be added.
  - Fluoxetine (Prozac), an antidepressant
- Benzodiazepines can be used for acute anxiety.

© 2014 American Nurses Credentialing Center

ADHD: Management of Inattentive, Impulsive, and Hyperactive Types

333

- Medication management plus behavioral treatment.
- Medication algorithm
  - First-line
    - Psychostimulants make more DA and/or NE available.
  - Second-line
    - Antidepressants make more 5HT, DA, and NE available.
  - Third-line
    - Antihypertensives (alpha-2 agonists): Clonidine (Catapres) or guanfacine (Tenex). May be first-line for patients with ADHD and tics.

© 2014 American Nurses Credentialing Center

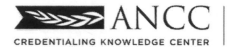
ADHD: Psychostimulants and Adjuncts

334

- Tailor the release characteristics to patient need
  - Immediate release compounds last 2 to 4 hours
  - Older sustained release compounds last about 4 hours
  - Newer sustained release offer longer coverage
    - Methylphenidate (Ritalin LA 8-12 hrs, Concerta 12 hrs, Daytrana (patch), Metadate CD 8 hrs, Quillivant XR)
    - lisdexamfetamine dimesylate (Vyvanse) 10 hours
    - Dextroamphetamine (Adderall XR): 9 hours
    - Dextroamphetamine (Dexedrine Spansule): 6-9 hours
    - Dexmethylphenidate (Focalin XR)
    - Atomoxetine (Strattera) – 1st non-stimulant, an SNRI
    - Guanfacine (Intuniv): Alpha-2A agonist, adjunct to stimulants

© 2014 American Nurses Credentialing Center

ADHD: Psychostimulants (cont.)

335

- Monitor: ECG baseline, BP, weight and height. Periodic monitoring of CBC, platelets, liver function, and ECG.

- "Drug holidays" may be offered during summer months to allow catch up from growth suppression.

© 2014 American Nurses Credentialing Center

Considerations for Children and Adolescents

336

- Diagnoses can be atypical, constantly change, are comorbid with other psychiatric disorders.

- Be aware of psychosocial aspects related to drug taking.

- Children have greater hepatic capacity, more glomerular filtration and less fatty tissue.
  - Lowered ability to store medications in fat results in quicker elimination and shorter half-lives.

© 2014 American Nurses Credentialing Center

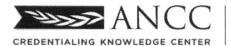
Implementations: Substance Use

337

- Detoxification initially
  - Safe and supportive environment
  - Lab tests, vital signs WNL
  - CIWA, COWS management
  - Pharmacology

- Rehabilitation
  - Peer support groups (AA, NA, AL-Anon, Al-A-Teen)
  - Relapse prevention strategies
  - Harm reduction strategies

© 2014 American Nurses Credentialing Center

Medication Management of Addictions

338

- Buprenorphine (Subutex): Semi-synthetic opioid used to treat opioid dependence: Ceiling effect reduces risk of overdose is less likely to cause respiratory depression
- Buprenorphine and naloxone (Suboxone): Semi-synthetic opioid used to treat opioid dependence
- Naloxone (Narcan): Opioid antagonist; reverses the effects of opioids
  - EMTs carry; new policy for community/public access.
- Naltrexone (Revia): Opioid antagonist; reverses the effects of opioids and alcohol
- Bupropion (Wellbutrin; Zyban): Smoking cessation aid.
- BZDPs: Alcohol/BZDP withdrawal
- Methadone: Maintenance therapy

© 2014 American Nurses Credentialing Center

Implementations: Eating Disorders

339

- Hospitalization may be indicated
- Nutritional stabilization with consult
- Help patient become aware of:
  - Cues that trigger problem eating responses
  - Thoughts, feelings, and assumptions associated with cues
  - Connections.
- Individual and family counseling

© 2014 American Nurses Credentialing Center

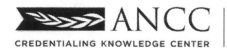
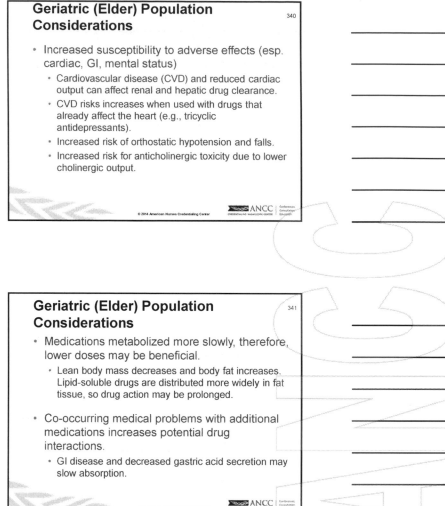

Geriatric (Elder) Population Considerations

340

- Increased susceptibility to adverse effects (esp. cardiac, GI, mental status)
  - Cardiovascular disease (CVD) and reduced cardiac output can affect renal and hepatic drug clearance.
  - CVD risks increases when used with drugs that already affect the heart (e.g., tricyclic antidepressants).
  - Increased risk of orthostatic hypotension and falls.
  - Increased risk for anticholinergic toxicity due to lower cholinergic output.

© 2014 American Nurses Credentialing Center

Geriatric (Elder) Population Considerations

341

- Medications metabolized more slowly, therefore, lower doses may be beneficial.
  - Lean body mass decreases and body fat increases. Lipid-soluble drugs are distributed more widely in fat tissue, so drug action may be prolonged.

- Co-occurring medical problems with additional medications increases potential drug interactions.
  - GI disease and decreased gastric acid secretion may slow absorption.

© 2014 American Nurses Credentialing Center

Implementations: Falls

342

- Strategies: Prevention!!
  - Reduce or eliminate hazards.
  - Install protective flooring.
  - Eliminate restraints and restraint hazards.
  - Increase staffing; place on close observation.
  - Monitor vital signs; orthostatic and any time a medication is changed, or added.
  - Increased attention if on diuretics; is a smoker; is confused or disoriented.
  - Enlist environmental safeguards, such as video monitoring, bed alarms.

© 2014 American Nurses Credentialing Center

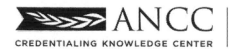
Implementations: Cognitive Disorders

343

- Address issues related to safety first!
  - Remove safety hazards.
  - Monitor behavioral changes/mental symptoms.
  - Supervise medications; neuroleptic medications if psychotic.
  - Restraints (only if necessary for safety) and one on one observation if hyperactive.
- Address basic biological needs:
  - Monitor vital signs
  - Adequate nutrition, food, fluid; adequate hydration
  - Help with hygiene, bathing, ADLs.

Implementations: Cognitive Disorders

344

- Address issues related to dependence
  - Provide reality orientation.
  - Provide structure and consistency, decrease stimulation.
  - Offer opportunity to participate and make choices when possible.
  - Communicate clearly and in simplistic form, keeping in mind memory problems.
  - Explain procedures, help with reality testing, reorient, decrease stimulation.
- Help caregivers cope
  - Provide help with care planning, education and grief/loss.

Managing Dementia

345

- Initiation
  - Start low and go slow; use psychopharm with care. Be alert to potential greater sensitivity to medication side effects and the impact of general medical conditions.
  - Initiate medication for enhancing cognitive functioning based on severity of symptoms.
  - Treat psychosis and agitation pharmacologically when such behavior is dangerous or upsetting.
  - Treat depression.
  - Some evidence for adding Vitamin E (2000/IU/day). Some evidence of increased risk of prostate cancer with use.
  - Educate caregivers.
- Stabilization and maintenance
  - Alzheimer's dementia is progressive, so needs will continually need to be reassessed.

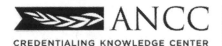
Medication Management of Dementia

346

- Mild to moderate Alzheimer Disease
  - Cholinesterase inhibitors make more ACh available. Treat the behavioral, psychological, and cognitive symptoms.
    - Adverse effects include nausea, diarrhea, vomiting, appetite loss, and increased gastric acid secretion.
      - Donepezil (Aricept): 5 to 10mg at night with slow titration
      - Tacrine (Cognex): 40 to 160mg/day
      - Rivastigmine (Exelon): 12 mg/day
      - Galantamine (Razadyne): 4 to 24 mg/day

Medication Management of Dementia

347

- Severe Alzheimer Disease
  - NMDA glutamate receptor antagonism stabilizes neurodegenerative process
    - Well tolerated; low incidence of adverse effects
      - Memantine (Namenda): 20 mg bid

- Coconut oil and Vitamin E are focus of current research.

Medication Management of Insomnia

348

- Physical and psychological dependence potential
  - Zolpidem tartrate (Ambien)
  - Zolpidem tartrate (Intermezzo) sublingual
  - Triazolam (Halcion)
  - Temazepam (Restoril)
  - Eszopiclone (Lunesta)

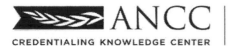
Medication Management of Aggressive Behavior: Options

349

- Goal: Prevent potential escalation of aggression to assault!
- Antipsychotics / Neuroleptics / Major Tranquilizers
- Mood Stabilizers / Anticonvulsants
- Antidepressants
- Lithium
- Antianxiety / Anxiolytics / Minor Tranquilizers (benzodiazepines)
- Propranolol (Inderal)

Behavioral Management: Aggression

350

- Maintain safety: Observe for escalation.
- Remain calm: Defuse with least restrictive means.
- De-escalation techniques and communication strategies
  - Speak in a calm, low voice. Use "I" language, don't take personally and avoid intense eye contact.
  - Respect need for personal space.
  - Acknowledge patient's feelings; reassure that staff are there to help.
  - Clearly communicate patient behavior and expected behavior. Ask "what do you need?" focus on disruptive behavior, not "bad patient."
- Environmental strategies
  - Structure the milieu with opportunities for less stimulation.
  - Offer opportunity for time out.
  - Always use least restrictive interventions.
  - Seclusion and restraints as a last resort.

Implementations: Suicidal or Homicidal Ideation

351

- A high-priority role for the professional RN:
  - Establish trust, rapport.
  - Determine suicide/homicide risk:
    - If risk is high, hospitalize.
    - Place on constant 1.1 monitoring.
    - Identify plan, means, lethality (remove lethal items).
  - Plan for psychopharmacology.
  - Engage in a discussion of current crisis.
  - Engage in work on an individualized crisis/safety plan.
  - Identify supports.
  - Psychoeducation to family, friends.
    - Suicide hotlines.
    - Community support groups.

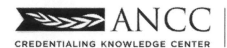
Implementations: Pain Management

352

- Prioritize interventions based on level of pain.
- Medication management
  - Opioids, benzodiazepines: Dependence/abuse potential
  - Medications that do not cause dependence
    - Non-steroidal anti-inflammatories (NSAIDs), Tricyclic antidepressants (TCAs), Selective Serotonin Reuptake Inhibitors (SSRIs), Selective Norepinephrine Reuptake Inhibitors (SNRIs), Anticonvulsants, Corticosteroids
- Provide skills/knowledge to facilitate understanding for appropriate and safe management
- Teach alternative pain management skills
  - Distraction, guided imagery
  - Gentle exercise (yoga, deep breathing)
  - Relaxing music
  - Biofeedback, cognitive coping skills

© 2014 American Nurses Credentialing Center

Implementations: Sleep Hygiene and Promotion

353

- Remove or treat underlying causes.
  - Assessment may include polysomnography.
- Rise at same time each day; Avoid daytime napping.
  - Maintain comfortable sleeping conditions; spend no longer than 20 minutes awake in bed; adjust sleep hours and routine to optimize daily schedule and living situation.
- Engage in calming activities at night (e.g., bath, relaxation).
  - Avoid evening stimulation (e.g., TV); establish physical fitness habits earlier in day.
- Eat on regular schedule; light at night.
- Discontinue use of drugs that act on CNS.
  - Sedative-hypnotics or benzodiazepines may be used for short periods (<7 to 10 days up to 2 months) to promote sleep; may be continued 2 to 3 nights per week for refractory insomnia.
- Adapted from Keltner & Folks, 2005

© 2014 American Nurses Credentialing Center

Implementations with Communication and Language Deficits

354

- Identify barriers to compliance, (i.e., hearing/visual/cognitive/developmental deficits.)
- Use the same sequence and repeat phrases.
- Speak slowly and clearly; use simple sentences.
- Encourage by listening, smiling, use of pictures and gestures.
- Allow time for translation and processing.
- Help patient develop realistic, culturally relevant goals.
- Incorporate cultural-specific teaching formats.

© 2014 American Nurses Credentialing Center

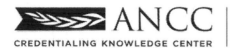

Implementations: Gender Dysphoria 355

- Counseling for social transitioning
- Cross-sex hormone therapy (estrogens, testosterones)
- Gender reassignment surgery
- Legal advice
- Health insurance: Current ethical issue (are mammograms covered when performed on males transgendered to females, etc.)
- Advocacy: Stigma elimination

© 2014 American Nurses Credentialing Center

005: Pharmacological, Biological, & Integrative Therapies (Part 2)

Session 005: Learning Objectives 357

1. Discuss nurse-initiated and collaborative strategies related to the implementation of somatic, complementary and integrative treatments for improved patient outcomes.
2. Discuss the management of crises in guiding seclusion and restraint decisions.

© 2014 American Nurses Credentialing Center

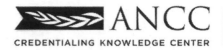

SOMATIC, COMPLEMENTARY, ALTERNATIVE, AND INTEGRATIVE THERAPIES

358

Somatic Treatment: Electroconvulsant Therapy (ECT)

359

- Therapeutic (clinically purposeful) induction of a unilateral or bilateral generalized seizure.
- Not a first-line treatment: Invasive; side effects:
  - Generally safe and effective in patients who have failed medication trials (up to 70% respond positively) or who have severe or psychotic symptoms, are acutely suicidal or homicidal, or have marked symptoms of agitation or stupor.
  - Fastest and most effective available therapy for major depression with or without psychosis, bipolar disorder, schizoaffective disorder, NMS, dementia with underlying mood disorder.

ECT Pre-Procedure Nursing Care

360

- Informed consent:
  - Explain and document consent related to beneficial and adverse effects, alternative treatments, natural course of the disorder, and option of no treatment.
- NPO six hours prior to treatment.
- Remove dentures or anything in mouth.
- Establish IV line.
- Insert bite block just before treatment.
- Administer 100% O2 at 5L per minute during procedure and until spontaneous respiration returns.

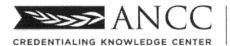
ECT Treatment Series
361

- Acute series: Treat disorder and restore functioning
  - 3 times a week
  - Typically 6-12 treatments
  - Improvements may be seen after 4-6 treatments
- Maintenance series: Maintains gains
  - May be weekly or monthly treatments
  - Can reduce or prevent inpatient stays
- Personal Account: The Man with the Electrofried Brain published 2013

© 2014 American Nurses Credentialing Center

ECT Induction, Mechanisms, Procedure
362

- Affects virtually every neurotransmitter system in the brain. Effects resemble changes that occur with antidepressants.
- Anticholinergics minimize oral and respiratory secretions.
- Anesthesia.
- Muscle relaxants minimize risk of bone fractures or injuries.
- EEG monitored for appearance of high-voltage delta and theta waves.

- Tonic/clonic seizure induced for 30-60 seconds. BP cuff may be kept inflated on one calf to observe seizure activity (fasciculation) distal to cuff.

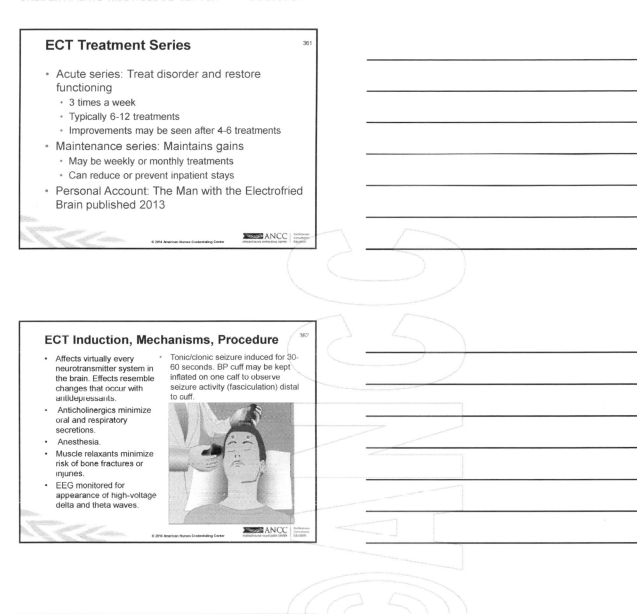

© 2014 American Nurses Credentialing Center

ECT Post-Procedure Nursing Care
363

- Monitor vital signs and O2 saturation with pulse oximetry upon return to unit and at 15 minute intervals.
- Observe mental status for common side effects:
  - Confusion, disorientation, headache, muscle aches and memory loss (temporary and reversible).
- After return of gag reflex, patient may resume eating meals.
- Reassure patient that most memory problems will resolve within several weeks.

© 2014 American Nurses Credentialing Center

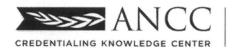

Somatic Treatment: Vagal Nerve Stimulation (VNS)

364

- Small wire (lead) device implanted under skin near collarbone.

- Vagus nerve stimulated with regular, mild pulses of electrical energy to the brain via the vagus nerve.

- Helpful with treatment-resistant depression.

Somatic Treatment: Deep Brain Stimulation (DBS)

365

- Surgical implantation of "brain pacemaker" which sends electrical impulses to select regions of the brain.
- Originally designed to treat Parkinson's disease, clinical trials show benefit for treatment of severe forms of treatment resistant depression an essential tremors, dystonia, and chronic pain.

Somatic Treatment: Transmagnetic Stimulation (rTMS)

366

- Noninvasive method causes depolarization or hyperpolarization of brain neurons.
- Uses electromagnetic induction to induce rapidly changing currents through a coil of wire applied near the head.
- Technique modulates activity of neurons.

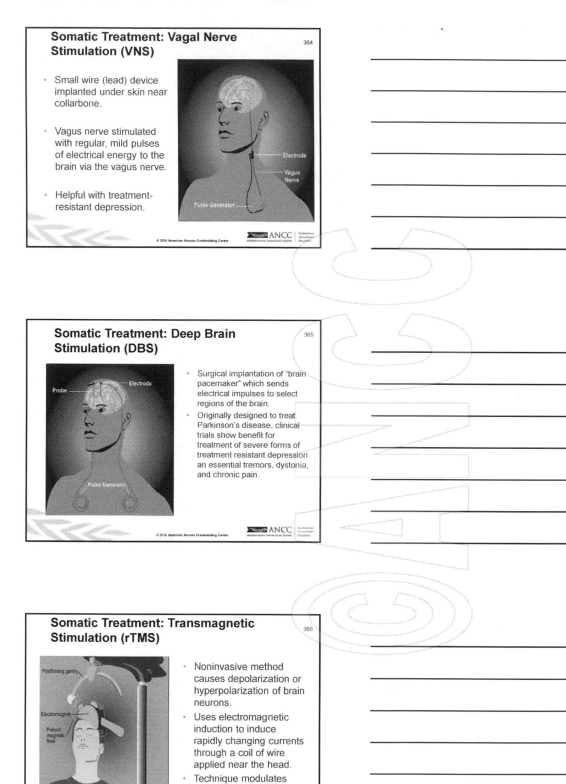

Somatic Therapy: Phototherapy

367

- Phototherapy is a portable lighting device known as a light box that may be prescribed primarily to treat Seasonal Affective Disorder (SAD), a mood disorder that presents in the winter months.
- The bright light therapy, administered at home, may act to readjust the body's circadian (daily) rhythms or internal clock.
- Phototherapy may also trigger the production of serotonin and melatonin.

© 2014 American Nurses Credentialing Center

ANCC

Complementary, Alternative, and Integrative Therapies

368

- Approximately 40% of Americans use complementary and integrative therapies
- Cover a broad range of healing philosophies, approaches, and therapies
  - Complementary and integrative therapies are used in addition to traditional medical practices.
  - Alternative therapies are used in place of traditional medical practices.

© 2014 American Nurses Credentialing Center

ANCC

Complementary, Alternative, and Integrative Therapies: Mind/Body Practices

369

- Biofeedback
- Heart Math Systems
- Yoga
- Meditation
- Guided imagery
- Phototherapy
- Therapeutic Touch
- Animal-assisted therapy
- Electroacupuncture

- Hypnotherapy (Hypnosis)
- Sound/music therapy
- Prayer
- Acupuncture
- Aromatherapy
- Ambient therapy
- Herbal preparations
- Expressive/creative art and music therapy

© 2014 American Nurses Credentialing Center

ANCC

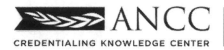
Biofeedback and HeartMath Systems

370

- Instruments that monitor and feed back moment to moment changes in physiology. Heart Math is computer generated.

- The individual perceives the information and learns to self-regulate.

- Control develops that ultimately eliminates the need for biofeedback.

© 2014 American Nurses Credentialing Center

Evaluation: Practice Standard 6

371

- Professional RN:
  - Evaluates patient response to all nursing interventions and identifies the degree to which patient goals and outcomes were achieved.
  - Applies nursing knowledge to determine the need to revise, modify, add, or discontinue patient problems, diagnoses and interventions.
    - Scores on standardized scales and screening tools
    - Physical exam and mental status
    - Laboratory and radiologic results
    - Medication response
  - Collaborates with patient, team, family, significant others to modify the plan of care (considering cultural beliefs, financial resources, community supports).

© 2014 American Nurses Credentialing Center

Evaluation of Pain Management Implementations

372

- Reassess signs and symptoms of pain response.
  - Use of 10 pt. scale or other standardized measurement.
- Evaluate family and friend observations.
- Continue to observe patient behaviors.

© 2014 American Nurses Credentialing Center

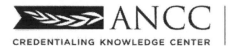
Evaluation: Pain Response

373

- **The patient:**
  - Has not experienced injury.
  - Accepted diagnosis.
  - Socialized appropriately.
  - Understood importance of medication adherence.
  - Improved with medication regimen.
  - Gained or nearly regained previous or optimal level of physical functioning.
  - Exhibited improved cognition.
  - Acknowledged problems and personal responsibility.
  - Used adaptive coping mechanism when stressed.
  - Ate well balanced meals.
  - Obtained adequate rest.
  - Patient/family gained education.
  - Participated in treatment planning.
  - Was willing to follow through on treatment plan.
  - Gained improved relationships with family/significant others.

© 2014 American Nurses Credentialing Center

374

CRISIS MANAGEMENT, AND SECLUSION/RESTRAINT

© 2014 American Nurses Credentialing Center

Crisis Concepts

375

- A crisis is a normal response or reaction to an overwhelming, traumatic event.
- Occurs when one's usual ways of coping are inadequate to deal with a stressor; homeostasis is disrupted; person unable to reestablish homeostasis resulting in functional impairment.
- May result in somatic complaints, perceptual changes, intense feelings, impulsivity and limited ability to ask for help.
- Crises are typically self-limiting and last from four to six weeks; most resolve within 72 hours without intervention.
- Maximum goal is improvement of functioning above pre-crisis level

© 2014 American Nurses Credentialing Center

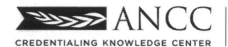
Types of Crises as Stressors

376

- Situational
  - Usually unplanned
  - Specific external event upsets the equilibrium

- Maturational
  - Can be planned for
  - Developmental events requiring role changes

- Adventitious (Global)
  - Unexpected disasters, accidents, or trauma
  - Usually causes more far-reaching destruction

© 2014 American Nurses Credentialing Center

Crisis Characteristics

377

- Persons experiencing a crisis may:
  - Display intense emotions: shock, confusion, anxiety.
  - Experience perceptual changes and intense feelings.
  - Utilize adaptive (e.g., denial) and maladaptive (e.g., heroic) defenses.
  - Show a decline in overall functioning or school performance.
  - Develop somatic complaints.
  - Display impaired impulse control.
  - Be isolated from usual supports.
  - Experience survivor guilt.

© 2014 American Nurses Credentialing Center

Phases of Crisis Intervention

378

1. Develop an alliance.
   - Build trust and utilize empathy.
   - Begin where the person wants.
   - Acknowledge helplessness.
2. Gather information.
   - Focus on precipitating event.
     - It may not be therapeutic to describe a traumatic event in detail.
     - Gather timeline and precipitating events.
   - Determine pre-crisis level of functioning.
     - Review similar past symptoms.
   - Determine acute and long-term needs, threats, and challenges.
   - Review past successful coping mechanisms.
   - Identify usual resources.

© 2014 American Nurses Credentialing Center

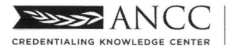
Phases of Crisis Intervention (cont.)

379

3. Problem-solving
   * Begin basic problem solving.
   * Set realistic goals.
   * Focus on termination from beginning.
   * Support positive strengths.
   * Suggest additional coping strategies.
4. Evaluation
   * Have identified outcomes been achieved?
   * Are adequate support systems in place?

© 2014 American Nurses Credentialing Center

Implementations: Crisis

380

* Implementations focus on triggers, feelings, and environmental monitoring.
* Basic physical needs:
  * Attend to emergencies.
  * Refer or link to social services.
* Basic psychological needs:
  * Listen, give support, support adaptive defenses, provide structure, encourage constructive activity.
  * Encourage preferred coping mechanisms.
  * Teach simple techniques for reducing stress.
  * Support previous successes and beliefs in self-efficacy.
  * Assist in setting up new supports or activating those already available.

© 2014 American Nurses Credentialing Center

Crisis Intervention: Seclusion or Restraints

381

* Basic right to treatment in the least restrictive setting.
* Standards for use regulated by TJC and CMS:
  * Must be therapeutically indicated and justified.
  * Reduction and/or elimination is new mandate.
* Standards to use:
  * When preventive and anticipatory strategies have failed.
  * Emergency situations presenting immediate risk of harm or safety to patient, staff, or others.
  * As a last resort when other methods have failed.
  * Standards for MD or LIP:
  * Patient evaluated within 1 hour of seclusion or restraint use.
  * Time-limited: Four hours for adults; Two hours for adolescents/children (9 to 17); One hour for children younger than 9; Therapeutic hold for children.

© 2014 American Nurses Credentialing Center

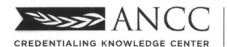
Seclusion and Restraint Team Response

382

- Intervene early in escalation process; allow patient least restrictive options (redirect to room, time out).
- If least restrictive measures fail, nurse communicates intent, and how it can help.
- Seclusion offered as first step.
- If necessary, notify security, obtain team assistance.
- Remove all others from the area.
- Leader express concern for the patient's safety and behavior.
- At given signal, team secures the patient's limbs.
- Escort patient to appropriate room or location communicate intent for seclusion and/or restraints.

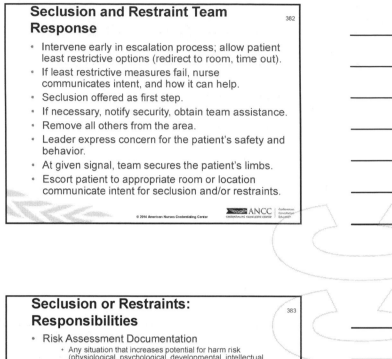

Seclusion or Restraints: Responsibilities

383

- Risk Assessment Documentation
  - Any situation that increases potential for harm risk (physiological, psychological, developmental, intellectual condition; spiritual distress).
  - Use standardized assessment tools when possible.
- Patient Care Documentation
  - Patient preferences to type of restraint (alternatives offered: time-out period). Use only minimum necessary for safety.
  - Medications administered if necessary.
  - Continuous/ongoing assessment, monitoring, reevaluation; document all behaviors, range of motion, circulation checks, vital signs.
  - Offer food/fluids, toileting, hygiene.
  - Notification to family of need for restraint intervention.
  - Terminate as soon as criteria for release is met.

Seclusion or Restraints: Responsibilities

384

- Documentation Components:
  - Document that risk was assessed.
  - Least restrictive options tried without success.
  - Description of the event (triggers?); rationale for use.
  - Patient response/behavior.
  - Patient's physical condition.
  - Nursing care that was provided.
  - Rationale for terminating the intervention.
  - Debriefing with patient, patient's, and staff to identify triggers to loss of control, options for alternatives that can be used in the future, barriers to providing least restrictive interventions.
- Legal assumption: Not documented, Not done!

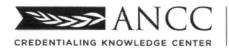

Review Question

385

The nurse on the disaster management team is observing that a survivor of the recent earthquake, who has lost all possessions, appears to be offering consolation and support to other affected community members. The nurse overhears the victim state to other survivors, "I have been through some other difficulties in life; we have our lives and each other. That's what's most important at this very moment." The nurse's best understanding of this behavior is that this person is:

a) Totally in shock, disbelief, denial.
b) Demonstrating resilience and coping abilities.
c) Functioning in the alarm stage of the general adaptation stage.
d) Staving off an inevitable breakdown by disassociating from this tragedy.

Review Question

386

During the treatment team's discharge planning meeting, the nurse reviews Johnny's medical record and notes the following: WBC 7,000, Sodium 143 mEq/L, HbA1c 6%, B/P 138/88, Lithium level 0.8 mEq/L, T 100.9, BUN 10 mg/dL, (carbamazepine) Tegretol level 100 mg/L, thrombocytes 200,000/mm3. What essential action should the nurse take prior to Johnny's discharge?

a) Report to the team that the carbamazepine (Tegretol) level is outside therapeutic levels.
b) Inform the team that blood chemistries and electrolytes are concerning.
c) Support the decision for discharge since his biopsychosocial outcomes seem stabilized.
d) Notify that patient that he will likely need referral to a urologist.

CATEGORY III: NURSE-PATIENT RELATIONSHIP, PROFESSIONAL DEVELOPMENT, AND LEADERSHIP

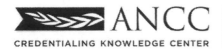

Conferences.
Consultation.
Education.

CATEGORY III A: NURSE-PATIENT
RELATIONSHIP

BEING THERAPEUTIC: CULTURAL
SENSITIVITY IN RELATIONSHIPS
AND IN COMMUNICATION

© 2014 American Nurses Credentialing Center

**006: Nurse-Patient Relationships,
Professional Development, &
Leadership (Part 1)**

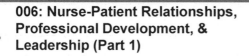

006: Learning Objectives   390

1. Discuss the role of the professional nurse in
   fostering and maintaining a therapeutic
   relationship with patients from differing cultural
   backgrounds across the life span.

2. Identify responsibilities and behaviors of the
   professional registered nurse in demonstrating
   accountability to self and to patient and family
   care in complex health care settings.

© 2014 American Nurses Credentialing Center

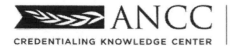

Conferences.
Consultation.
Education.

Critical Areas: Nurse-Patient Relationship 391

- Communication: culturally sensitive and professional.
  - Patient.
  - Patient care provider.
  - Health care team.
- Responsibilities of Professional Nurse:
  - Safety.
  - Quality.
  - Evidence-based practice.
  - Continued competence.
- Decision-Making at the Point of Care:
  - Prioritizing.
  - Delegating.
  - Patient satisfaction.
  - Time management.

© 2014 American Nurses Credentialing Center

Culture 392

- "The integrated pattern of human behavior that includes thoughts, communications, actions, customs, beliefs, values, and institutions of a racial, ethnic, religious, or social group." (Cross, 1989).

- Differences within cultures include: age, gender, sexual orientation, religion, spirituality, social class, education, occupation, ability/disability.

- Ethnocentrism is belief in the superiority of one's own culture and lifestyle.

- Stereotyping is assuming all members of a group have the same characteristics.

© 2014 American Nurses Credentialing Center

Ethnicity and Race 393

- Ethnicity
  - Shared feelings or identity among individual groups, based on sharing of similar cultural patterns, values, beliefs, customs, and behaviors that create a common history.
- Race
  - A social construction based on physical markers, such as skin color, to identify group membership.
  - Races are not genetically definable categories.
  - Racism is real and is related to social inequities.
  - Minorities (people of color) are more likely to receive lower-quality health care regardless of income and insurance coverage.

© 2014 American Nurses Credentialing Center
- IOM, 2002

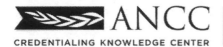
Cultural Competency

394

- "The ability to view each patient as a unique individual, fully considering the patient's cultural experiences within the context of the common developmental challenges faced by all people" (Stuart and Laria, 2005).
- Each person is first an individual and second, a member of a cultural or ethnic group.
- Developing cultural competence…
  - Be aware and willing to become sensitive (sensitivity).
  - Gain knowledge of cultural differences.
  - Learn skills in how to assess values, beliefs, practices.
  - Engage in cross-cultural interactions/encounters.
  - Have a desire to provide culturally competent care.

© 2014 American Nurses Credentialing Center

Developing Cultural Sensitivity

395

- Examine own communication
  - Stop using offensive language.
  - Respect patterns of communication.
  - Stop speaking in ways that are disrespectful of a person's cultural beliefs.
    - LEARN: (Campinha-Bacote, 1992)
  - Listen with empathy
  - Explain your perception of the patient's problem
  - Acknowledge similarities and differences in perceptions
  - Recommend treatment
  - Negotiate treatment
  - ** Get an interpreter!!

© 2014 American Nurses Credentialing Center

Assessment of Cultural Identity

396

- How does the individual identify himself/herself?

- Consider acculturation/immigration
  - Affinity of the person to the native culture or to the host culture.

- Native language: abilities and preferences.
  - Is English the 2nd language? (ESL)

- Cultural interpretation of functional levels.

© 2014 American Nurses Credentialing Center

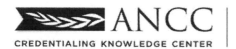
Areas for Cultural Assessment

397

- Family roles and social customs
- Preferred language
- Religious and spiritual beliefs and practices
- Rituals/practices around death, dying, and birth
- Social class distinctions
- Health practices and beliefs
- Dietary practices and rituals
- Physical space needs
- Sexual orientation (LGBTQI); Gender Identity
- Affective expression
- Meaning of nonverbal gestures and vocal quality

© 2014 American Nurses Credentialing Center

Areas for Cultural Sensitivity

398

- Risk Factors
  - Differences based on biology (genetics), economics, and environment.
- Etiquette/taboo regarding level of self disclosure
  - May feel offensive with certain questions.
- Space and Gender
  - Develop awareness of spatial needs and gender roles.
    - (e.g., Latinos and Africans have close personal space compared to Europeans and Asians).
- Time
  - Recognize cultural holidays and seasonal rituals of others.
  - Orientation may be towards future, past, present.
- Health, Illness, and Healers
  - May use nontraditional folk healers, acupuncture, herbalists, complementary and integrative techniques.

© 2014 American Nurses Credentialing Center

Areas for Cultural Sensitivity

399

- Families and Roles
  - Asians: Value and include older adults
  - Americans: Value youth
  - Africans, Latino(a)s, and Native Americans: value extended family
- Religious and Spiritual Beliefs
  - Europeans: Predominately Judeo-Christian
  - Asians: Taoism, Buddhism, Islam, or Christianity
  - Middle Easterners: Predominately Muslim
- Sexual Orientation
  - Be sensitive to LGBTQI needs
- Touch and Eye Contact

© 2014 American Nurses Credentialing Center

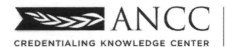
Culturally Sensitive Nursing Diagnoses and Planning

400

- Cultural factors affect
  - The expression, prevalence, and interpretation of assessment data and treatment options for mental disorders.
- NANDA related to cultural/spiritual problems
  - Impaired verbal communication, such as misinterpretation of dialect, thereby imposing own values to situation, person
  - Spiritual distress
- Planning
  - Consider social support system as well as beliefs in culturally traditional healthcare practices.

© 2014 American Nurses Credentialing Center

Culturally Sensitive Nursing Implementations and Evaluations

401

- Implementations
  - Obtain a skilled interpreter if necessary.
  - Assist patient/family in designing a therapeutic diet with preferred foods.
  - Enlist family members to assist with care if desired within the culture.
  - Allow patient to express fears, concerns, and distress; encourage religious rituals if appropriate.
- Evaluation
  - Based on achievement of expected outcomes from cultural perspective.

© 2014 American Nurses Credentialing Center

Therapeutic Relationship

402

- A mutual learning experience and a facilitating emotional and cognitive experience for the patient.
- Fosters goal attainment that support optimal growth outcomes.
  - Self-realization
  - Self-acceptance
  - Increased genuine self-respect
  - Ability to form interpersonal relationships
  - Improved functioning

© 2014 American Nurses Credentialing Center

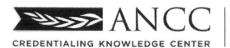
Interpersonal One-to-One Nurse-Patient Relationship (Peplau)

403

- Interpersonal processes
  - Significant and therapeutic (meaningful).
  - Learning situations that promote health and maximize capabilities.
- Essential nursing skills
  - Observation
  - Interpretation (listening skills)
  - Intervention
- Nurses are "participant observers" during the therapeutic process. Observe patient behavior and own behavior.

© 2014 American Nurses Credentialing Center

Interpersonal One-to-One Nurse-Patient Relationship (Peplau)

404

- Four phases of relationship development characterized by dynamic learning experience for both patient and nurse.
  - Orientation
    - Create environment for trust and rapport
    - Conduct assessment and data collection
    - Identify patient's strengths and limitations
    - Formulate nursing diagnoses.
  - Identification
    - Clarify expectations
    - Set mutually agreeable goals
    - Develop realistic plan of action.

© 2014 American Nurses Credentialing Center

Interpersonal One-to-One Nurse-Patient Relationship (Peplau)

405

- Exploitation (working phase)
  - Maintain trust and rapport
  - Promote patient's insight and perception of reality
  - Use problem-solving to work toward goals
  - Teach new skills
  - Confront supportively
  - Continuously evaluate progress toward goals.
- Termination
  - Facilitate closure of relationship
  - Identify progress toward goal attainment (nurse and patient perspectives)
  - Identify issues which need further work
  - Make necessary referrals
  - Recognize and explore feelings and thoughts about termination.

© 2014 American Nurses Credentialing Center

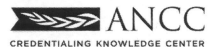

ANCC | Conferences.
Consultation.
Education.

CREDENTIALING KNOWLEDGE CENTER

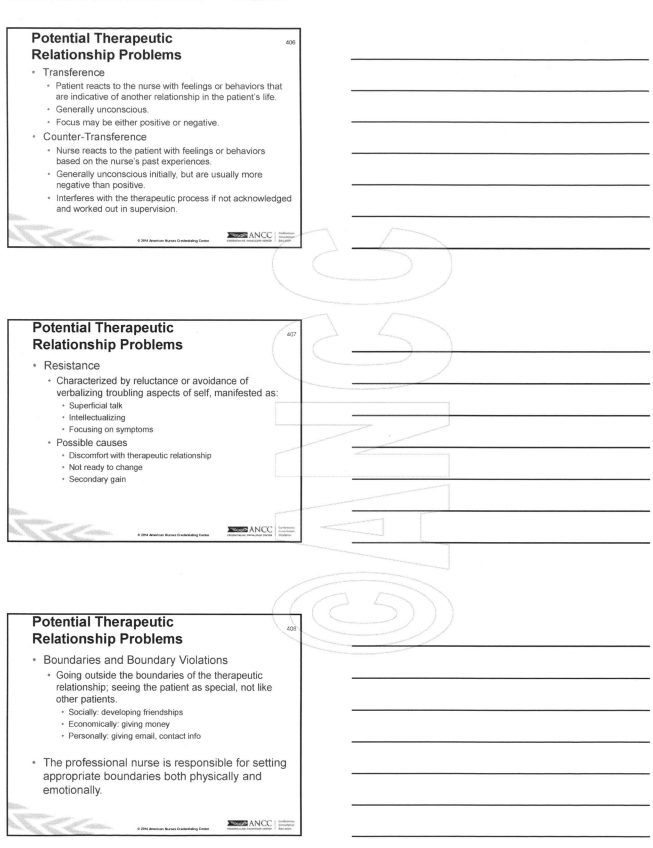

Potential Therapeutic Relationship Problems

406

- Transference
  - Patient reacts to the nurse with feelings or behaviors that are indicative of another relationship in the patient's life.
  - Generally unconscious.
  - Focus may be either positive or negative.
- Counter-Transference
  - Nurse reacts to the patient with feelings or behaviors based on the nurse's past experiences.
  - Generally unconscious initially, but are usually more negative than positive.
  - Interferes with the therapeutic process if not acknowledged and worked out in supervision.

© 2014 American Nurses Credentialing Center

Potential Therapeutic Relationship Problems

407

- Resistance
  - Characterized by reluctance or avoidance of verbalizing troubling aspects of self, manifested as:
    - Superficial talk
    - Intellectualizing
    - Focusing on symptoms
  - Possible causes
    - Discomfort with therapeutic relationship
    - Not ready to change
    - Secondary gain

© 2014 American Nurses Credentialing Center

Potential Therapeutic Relationship Problems

408

- Boundaries and Boundary Violations
  - Going outside the boundaries of the therapeutic relationship; seeing the patient as special, not like other patients.
    - Socially: developing friendships
    - Economically: giving money
    - Personally: giving email, contact info

- The professional nurse is responsible for setting appropriate boundaries both physically and emotionally.

© 2014 American Nurses Credentialing Center

Therapeutic Communication (Hildegard Peplau)

409

- Is responsive
  - Empathic, respectful, genuine, immediate attentiveness, warm, promotes reality-based exchanges
- Establishes trust, rapport, and openness
- Conveys support without supporting delusional thinking
  - "I understand that you believe you are the owner of this hospital, but I see it differently."
    - Built from authenticity (honesty), consistency, confidentiality
- Demonstrates respect for cultural differences
  - Is clear and easy to understand; considers verbal/non-verbal aspects
  - Confidentiality is assured
  - Confrontation is only used therapeutically

© 2014 American Nurses Credentialing Center

Therapeutic Communication Skills

410

- Empathy
- Active listening
- Use of silence
- Reflecting
- Imparting information
- Clarifying
- Paraphrasing
- Checking perceptions
- Questioning

- Structuring
- Pinpointing
- Linking
- Giving feedback
- Confronting
- Summarizing
- Processing
- Reframing

© 2014 American Nurses Credentialing Center

Therapeutic Communication: Interviewing

411

- Open-ended questions
  - Elicit the client's story: "What brings you here today?"
- Closed-ended questions
  - More fully describe and identify specific problems.
    - Can be answered with "yes" or "no."
- Communication skill examples
  - "Let's go over what we have accomplished so far."
    - Summarizing
  - "It sounds as though you are saying you have had enough."
    - Paraphrasing
  - "I'm not sure I understand what you mean."
    - Clarifying
  - "You feel guilty."
    - Reflecting

© 2014 American Nurses Credentialing Center

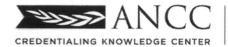
Non-Therapeutic Communication

412

- False reassurance
  - "You'll be fine."

- Giving advice
  - "You should get a job."

- False inferences
  - "You really don't like the idea of getting up and going to work each day."

- Moralizing
  - "Accepting food stamps is wrong when you are healthy."

- Value judgments
  - "She is a good patient."

- Social responses
  - "Oh well, that's just the way it goes."

© 2014 American Nurses Credentialing Center

Sources of Communication Problems

413

- Physical and cognitive impairments
  - (e.g., hearing, vision, literacy, cognition, memory)
- Language
  - Verbal: Culture, native language, vocal pitch/quality, tone, cadence, and rate.
  - Nonverbal: Body language, gender, and appearance.
- Culture
  - Different beliefs, norms, and values; stereotypes.
  - Affect perceptions of health/illness, help-seeking behavior, and outcomes.
- Non-therapeutic relationship

© 2014 American Nurses Credentialing Center

CATEGORY III B: PROFESSIONAL DEVELOPMENT

© 2014 American Nurses Credentialing Center

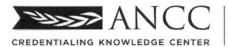
Education: Professional Performance Standard 8

415

- Maintaining competency
  - Knowledge building/continuing education
  - Patient encounters
  - Professional meetings
  - In-service programs, workshops, or courses
- Mentoring
- Precepting
- Role modeling
- Peer review/appraisals
- Specialty certifications

© 2014 American Nurses Credentialing Center

Nursing Practice Professionalism

416

- ANA's Social Policy Statement (2010)
  - Values and Assumptions
- Essential features of professional nursing
  - Attention to the full range of human experiences
  - Integration of objective data with knowledge
  - Application of scientific knowledge
  - Provision of a caring and facilitative relationship.
- Nursing scholars and theories
  - Concepts, principles, and processes that guide nursing observations, interpretations, and interventions
  - Frameworks that guide the nursing process
  - Refined through scholarly inquiry.

© 2014 American Nurses Credentialing Center

Major Nursing Theorists and Focus Areas

417

- Hildegard Peplau – Interpersonal One-to-One
- Dorothy Johnson – Behavioral Systems
- Madeline Leininger – Culture Care
- Dorothea Orem – Self Care
- Rosemarie Parse – Becoming
- Nola Pender – Health Promoting Lifestyle Behaviors
- Martha Rogers – Unitary Human Being
- Sister Callista Roy – Adaptation
- Jean Watson – Caring Science
- Gail Stuart – Stress Adaptation Model
- Ann Wolbert Burgess – Rape-Trauma Syndrome

© 2014 American Nurses Credentialing Center

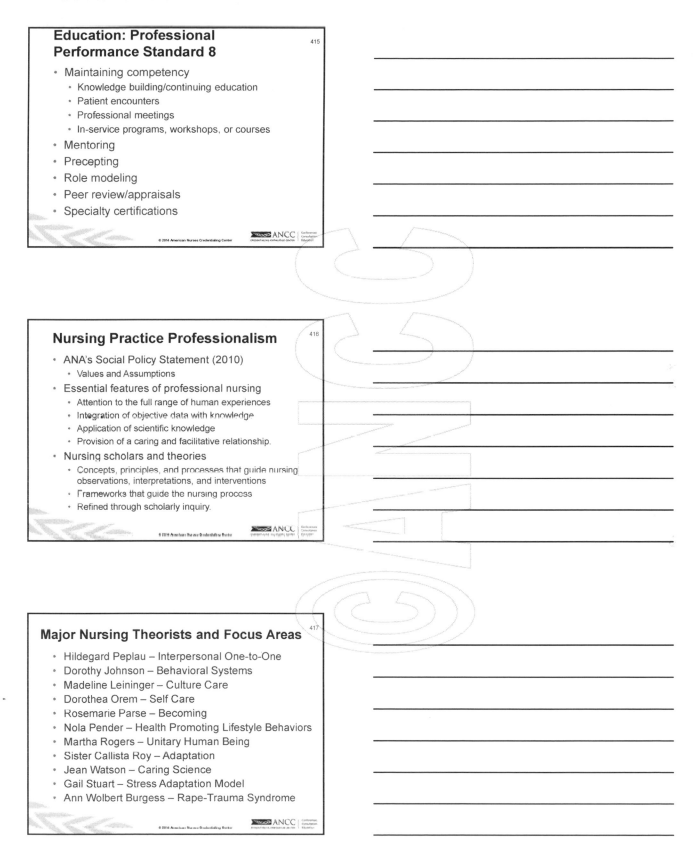

Professional Development Strategies

418

* Professional Nursing Organizations: Attend conferences
  * National League for Nursing (NLN)
  * American Nurses Association (ANA)
  * American Psychiatric Nurses Association (APNA)
    * (Policy Implications of Integrated Care – NEW)
  * International Society of Psychiatric Nurses (ISPN)
* Continuing education/continued competence
  * Read professional journals
  * Attend workshops, courses
  * Web-based resources, webinars
  * Examine trends in health care (SAMHSA, NIDA, NIMH, NCCAM, MHA, IOM, IHI, AHRQ)

© 2014 American Nurses Credentialing Center

Developing Presentation Skills

419

* PRACTICE…Just Do It!
  * Present patient cases and in-services
  * Present quality improvement data
  * Publish in nursing and other peer-reviewed journals
  * Develop portfolio, resume
  * Be interviewed
  * Engage in public speaking at church, conferences, schools

© 2014 American Nurses Credentialing Center

Research: Professional Performance Standard 13

420

* The professional RN integrates research findings into practice
  * Utilizes best available evidence, including research findings, to guide practice decisions
  * Actively participates in research activities at various levels appropriate to the nurse's level of education and position, including
    * Identification of clinical problems
    * Participation in data collection
    * Participation in formal committee
    * Sharing research findings with peers and others
    * Uses research findings in the development of policies, procedures, and standards of practice

© 2014 American Nurses Credentialing Center

Collaboration in Research Design, Implementation, and Utilization

421

* The professional RN collaborates (Professional Performance Standard 11) with others to enhance health care.
* This includes participation in research (Professional Performance Standard 13) and collaborative discussions to plan changes in care based on findings.
* After systematic search for best practices (Professional Performance Standard 14), the nurse collaborates with the patient and the interdisciplinary team to change the plan of care and evaluate outcomes.

© 2014 American Nurses Credentialing Center

Five Steps of Evidence-Based Practice

422

1. Ask an answerable clinical question.
   * Consider **PICO** in asking a relevant clinical question:
     * Patient population
     * Intervention or area of interest
     * Comparison interventions
     * Outcome measures
2. Collect the most relevant and best evidence.
3. Critically appraise the evidence.
4. Synthesize and integrate with professional experience, patient preferences, and values in making a practice decision or change.
5. Evaluate the practice decision or change.

© 2014 American Nurses Credentialing Center

Evidence-Based Sources: Seeking The "Gold Standard"

423

* Cochrane reviews.
* Agency for Healthcare Quality and Research (AHRQ). www.guidelines.gov
* Joanna Briggs Institute.
* Seek to identify
  * Systematic reviews of the literature
  * Review as many research studies as possible
  * Consider the best evidence hierarchy when evaluating the validity of the evidence
  * Search for best practice guidelines, clinical pathways
* (www.cochrane.org)

© 2014 American Nurses Credentialing Center

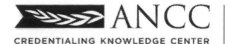

Best Evidence Hierarchy 424

- Meta-analyses (systematic reviews) of all randomized controlled trials (RCTs), or evidence-based clinical practice guidelines based on systematic reviews of RCTs
- RCTs considered the "Gold Standard" (Double-blinded RCT; Single RCT)
- Quasi-experimental controlled trials without randomization
- Case-control and cohort studies
- Systematic reviews of descriptive and qualitative studies
- Single descriptive or qualitative studies
- Opinions or reports of authorities or expert committees

© 2014 American Nurses Credentialing Center

Best Practice Models 425

- Broad consensus statements that integrate systems, providers, services, teams; Often used in inpatient settings and serve as a shortened version of the multidisciplinary care plan.
- Clinical Pathways are practice guidelines that identify key clinical processes and corresponding timelines;
  - Provide detailed specification of methods, treatment strategies, procedures, and interventions to ensure effective treatment.
  - Identifies target population based on diagnoses, conditions, treatments, interventions, or behaviors.
  - Documents patient care activities, variances, and goal achievement.
  - Expected outcome described in a measurable, realistic, and patient-centered way.
- Sources of practice guidelines based on diagnosis include:
  - American Psychiatric Nurses Association
  - National Guideline Clearinghouse
- Algorithms and Protocols
  - Specific sets of treatment based upon strongest evidence base.

© 2014 American Nurses Credentialing Center

Research vs. Outcome Evaluation 426

- Research: The systematic gathering of information to gain, expand, or validate knowledge about health and responses to health problems.
  - Research utilization: Use of research findings in practice settings.
- Outcome evaluation: Final activity of evidence-based practice that examines whether the application of evidence-based care resulted in an improvement or met expected treatment goals. What do the METRICS tell us?

© 2014 American Nurses Credentialing Center

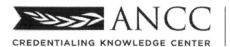
Qualitative Studies

427

- Research type that generally uses observation as the data collection method.
- Observation is the selection and recording of behaviors of people in their environment.
- Methods
  - Phenomenological
  - Grounded or Lived experiences

© 2014 American Nurses Credentialing Center

Quantitative Studies

428

- Research type that uses quantities, metrics, numbers to describe a phenomenon. Findings are described according to the strength of the numbers.
- Methods
  - Descriptive studies
    - Numerical values summarize, organize, and describe observations (mean, variance, standard deviation).
    - May be generated by either quantitative or qualitative research designs.
  - Inferential studies
    - Numerical values used to generalize about probabilities on the basis of a sample.
    - Can be used to test hypotheses.
    - Generated by quantitative research designs (analysis of variance, probability, probability value).

© 2014 American Nurses Credentialing Center

Descriptive Statistics

429

- Mean
  - Measure of central tendency derived by summing all scores and dividing by the number of participants.
- Variance
  - Measure of variation derived by squaring each deviation in a set of scores and then taking the mean of the squares. The larger the variance, the larger the dispersion of scores.
- Standard Deviation
  - Measure of variation derived by taking the square root of the variance. In a normal distribution, ±1SD includes 68% of the population; ±2 SD includes 95% of the population, and ± 3 SD includes 99% of the population.

© 2014 American Nurses Credentialing Center

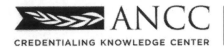
Inferential Statistics

430

- Analysis of Variance
  - Set of statistical procedures designed to compare two or more groups of observations. It determines whether the differences between groups are due to experimental influence or due to chance alone.
- Probability
  - Qualitative statement of the likelihood that an event will occur. A probability of 0 means that the event is certain not to occur; a probability of 1 means that the event will occur with certainty.
- Probability value (p value)
  - The probability of obtaining a result by chance alone. A p value of .01 means that the probability of obtaining a result by chance alone is one in 100; a p value of .05 means that the result will occur five times out of every 100 times by chance alone.

© 2014 American Nurses Credentialing Center

Critically Appraise Research Findings

431

- Sample size
- Significance
- Generalizability
- Use of control groups; randomization
- Did the study design match the question?
  - Treatment effects/randomized controlled trials
  - Prognosis/cohort study
  - Diagnosis/cross-sectional study
  - Lived experience/qualitative study
- Research finding conclusions "suggest" and do not "prove" anything.

© 2014 American Nurses Credentialing Center

Critically Appraise Research Findings

432

- Are the results valid?
  - Internal validity: Did the independent variable (treatment) result in a change in the dependent variable (outcome measure).
  - External validity: Is the sample representative of the population and can the results can be generalized to others? Was a power analysis used to determine sample size?
- Are the results reliable?
  - Reliability consistently and accurately measures the construct of interest.
- Are the results applicable?
  - Are the results appropriate and helpful to use in the setting and with the population of interest?
- Research results/findings/conclusions do not "prove" anything; they merely suggest by informing.

© 2014 American Nurses Credentialing Center

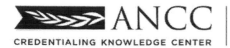
Ethics: Professional Performance Standard 12

433

- Principles or codes of conduct based on a person's understanding of right vs. wrong, proper, and moral.
  - An act can be:
    - Legal and ethical
    - Legal, but not ethical
    - Ethical, but not legal
    - Neither ethical nor legal
- Influenced by social understandings, family, religious and cultural standards, institutions, government.

© 2014 American Nurses Credentialing Center

Ethical Concepts and Approaches

434

- Justice
  - Fairness to everyone, sound reason, rightfulness of decisions and actions.
- Boneficence
  - The duty to do good, avoid harm to others.
- Nonmaleficence
  - The duty to do no harm to others.

- Fidelity
  - The duty to be true and loyal to others.
- Autonomy
  - The duty to protect the rights of a person to make decisions and take actions without external control.
- Veracity
  - The duty to tell the truth, and not to lie or deceive another.

- Approaches:
  - Utilitarianism: Do the ends justify the means?
  - Deontology: Are decisions absolute - right or wrong?

© 2014 American Nurses Credentialing Center

Research Ethics and Integrity

435

- Institutional Review Boards (IRBs) review all research studies to ensure that:
  - Risks to subjects are minimized
  - Subject selection is equitable
  - Informed consent (or assent) is obtained and documented
  - Data and safety monitoring plan is implemented when indicated
- All investigators or individuals involved in research studies must take and pass a required test on the Protection of Human Subjects based on the Belmont Report (1978).
  - Beneficence (do no harm)
  - Respect for human dignity (right for self-determination)
  - Justice (fair treatment and nondiscriminatory selection)

© 2014 American Nurses Credentialing Center

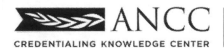
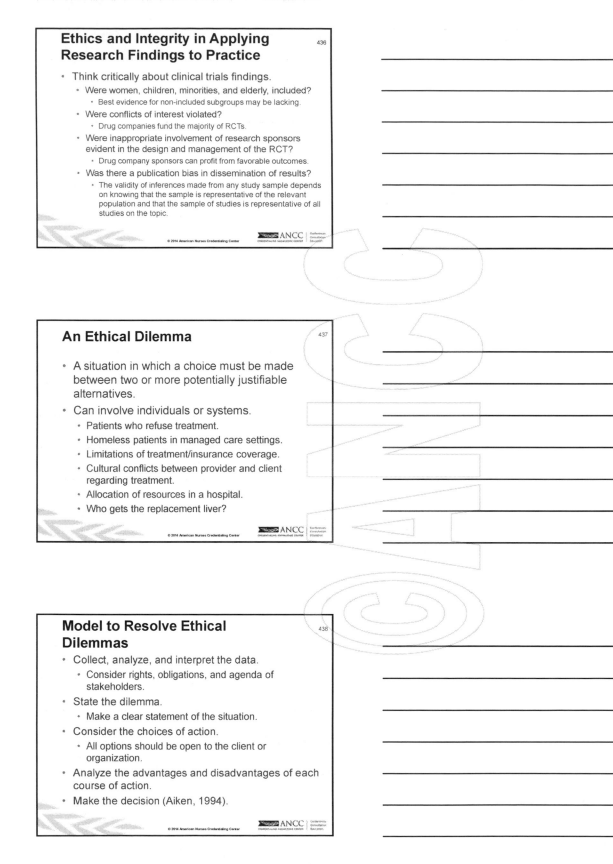

Ethics and Integrity in Applying Research Findings to Practice

436

- Think critically about clinical trials findings.
  - Were women, children, minorities, and elderly, included?
    - Best evidence for non-included subgroups may be lacking.
  - Were conflicts of interest violated?
    - Drug companies fund the majority of RCTs.
  - Were inappropriate involvement of research sponsors evident in the design and management of the RCT?
    - Drug company sponsors can profit from favorable outcomes.
  - Was there a publication bias in dissemination of results?
    - The validity of inferences made from any study sample depends on knowing that the sample is representative of the relevant population and that the sample of studies is representative of all studies on the topic.

An Ethical Dilemma

437

- A situation in which a choice must be made between two or more potentially justifiable alternatives.
- Can involve individuals or systems.
  - Patients who refuse treatment.
  - Homeless patients in managed care settings.
  - Limitations of treatment/insurance coverage.
  - Cultural conflicts between provider and client regarding treatment.
  - Allocation of resources in a hospital.
  - Who gets the replacement liver?

Model to Resolve Ethical Dilemmas

438

- Collect, analyze, and interpret the data.
  - Consider rights, obligations, and agenda of stakeholders.
- State the dilemma.
  - Make a clear statement of the situation.
- Consider the choices of action.
  - All options should be open to the client or organization.
- Analyze the advantages and disadvantages of each course of action.
- Make the decision (Aiken, 1994).

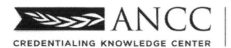

Conferences.
Consultation.
Education.

Ethical Responsibilities of Nurses

439

* Honor patient's confidentiality.
* Practice within area of expertise and competence.
* Maintain accurate records.
* Clarify nursing responsibilities to patients and families.
* Serve as a patient advocate.
* Maintain a therapeutic nurse/patient relationship.
* Demonstrate a commitment to self-care.
* Participate on committees that determine ethical outcomes for patients, organizations, and self.

© 2014 American Nurses Credentialing Center

Confidentiality

440

* An ethical concept that states that what is said between two people will not be shared elsewhere without consent.
* Legally regulated by the Health Insurance Portability and Accountability Act (HIPAA) of 2003.
  * Created to protect the privacy of individuals in the healthcare system.
  * Provides patients with access to their medical records and more control over how protected health information (PHI) is used and disclosed.

© 2014 American Nurses Credentialing Center

Exception to Confidentiality

441

* Protected health information (PHI) is considered confidential unless disclosure is required to prevent clear and imminent danger to the patient or others, and when legal requirements demand that confidential information be revealed.

* Electronic Health Records (EHR)
  * Clinical Decision Support

© 2014 American Nurses Credentialing Center

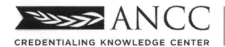
HIPAA Defines PHI

442

- Defines who may see or use health information and what they can do with it.
- Limits many uses and disclosures of health information to the "minimum necessary" amount needed for the task.
- Establishes new patient rights concerning their health information.
- Examples of PHI
  - Written information (reports, charts, letters, messages, etc.)
  - Oral communication (phone calls, meetings, informal conversations, etc.)
  - E-mail, computerized and electronic information (computer records, faxes, voicemail, PDA entries, etc.)

© 2014 American Nurses Credentialing Center

Maintaining PHI Records

443

- Use, and do not share computer passwords.
- Lock doors/file cabinets, and limit access to workspace where health information is used or stored.
- Limit access to printers and faxes where health information is printed.
- Limit access to health information to only those who need it for a specific task.
- Shred or otherwise properly dispose of health information.
- Use and keep only the minimum health information necessary for a specific task.
- Follow agency privacy policies and procedures.

© 2014 American Nurses Credentialing Center

Written Documentation and Charting

444

- Objective
- Subjective
- Interdisciplinary
- Restrictive measures
- Treatment plan/outcome documentation
- Risk assessment documentation
- Mental status
- Occurrence report

© 2014 American Nurses Credentialing Center

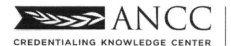
Problem-Oriented Documentation

445

- Chart note refers to the identified problem by name or number
- Changes are documented
  - Subjective
  - Objective
  - Assessment
  - Planning
  - Intervention
  - Evaluation

Focused Documentation

446

- Focus might be a sign or symptom, a nursing diagnosis, a behavior, a condition, a significant event, or an acute change in condition. It can be a positive focus, such as a patient strength.
  - Data: Includes S and O, behaviors, and status
  - Action: Includes plan and intervention
  - Response: Evaluation of response to interventions

Charting by Exception

447

- Flow sheets have pre-defined assessment and patient progress parameters based on written standards.
- Interdisciplinary team can chart by initialing that required interventions were provided.
- Abnormal or significant deviations are charted in descriptive format. When care was omitted, document action and rationale.
- Formats
  - Flow sheets
  - Clinical pathways

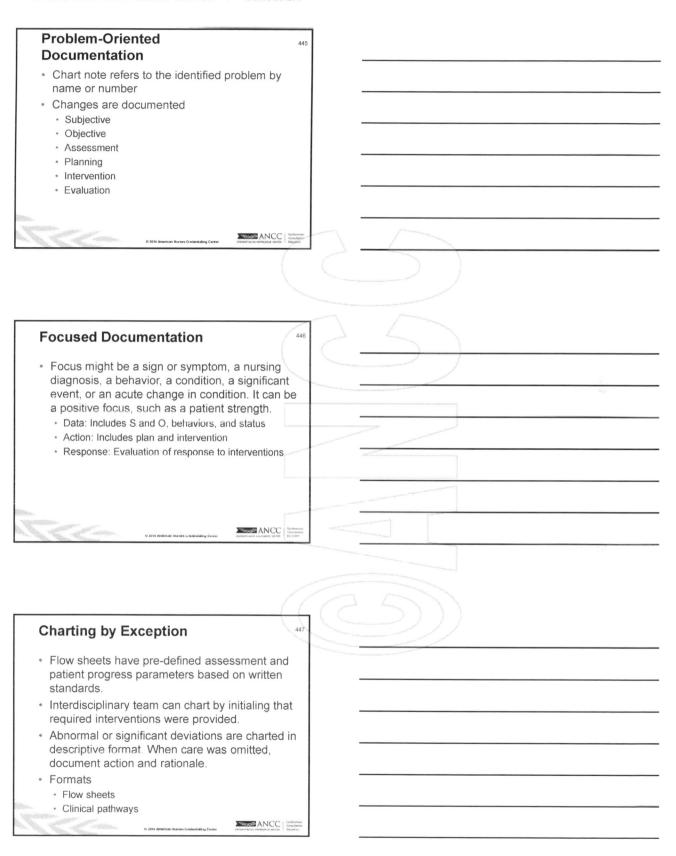

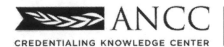
Occurrence Documentation

448

- Document occurrences when care or patient response is outside of expected norms which may affect patient quality and/or safety.
- Follow institutional policy and use appropriate forms.
- Examples
  - Sentinel events
  - Quality variances
  - Infectious disease
  - Medication errors
  - Patient harm

TJC Standards: Admission and Discharge

449

- Prior to admission
  - Identify and use information sources about patient needs.
  - Communicate with other care settings and organizations.
- During admission
  - Provide services consistent with clinic/hospital mission, population served, and setting.
  - Make arrangements with other organizations and settings to facilitate the patient's admission.
  - Reconcile medications and treatments across settings.
  - Patients are referred and transferred to meet their needs based on intensity, risk, and staffing levels.
  - When appropriate, clinical consultants and contractual arrangements are used for referrals and transfers.

TJC Standards: Admission and Discharge

450

- In the hospital
  - Services flow continuously from assessment through treatment and reassessment.
  - Patient care is individualized and coordinated between providers.
  - Age, developmental, and family-centered care is collaborated between, and delivered across the health care continuum.
- Before discharge
  - The need for discharge planning assessment is determined.
  - Education prepares the patient and family for discharge.
  - Understands early signs and symptoms of relapse and strategies to address issues (safety plan hotlines provider contacts).

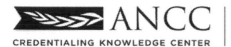
TJC Standards: Admission and Discharge

451

- At discharge
  - Patient needs are individualized and reassessed.
  - Patient is referred to providers, settings, resources, or organizations.
  - Hospital provides information or data to help others meet the patient's continuing aftercare needs.

Voluntary Admission

452

- In some states, voluntarily admitted patients can be detained 24 to 72 hours after submitting a discharge request.
- Short-term or observational hospitalization
  - For diagnosis and short-term therapy.
  - Patient agrees to receive treatment and abide by hospital rules.
  - Parent or legal guardian may request admission.
  - Patient retains all civil rights.
- Long-term hospitalization
  - For treatment, until determined ready for discharge.

Involuntary Admission

453

- Involuntary commitment is a legal process leading to "commitment" ("emergency petition," "50B," "5151" in CA, "pink slip").
  - Begins with a sworn petition
  - One or two MDs/LIPs must complete face-to-face examination
  - Person looses the right to leave the hospital when desired
  - Patient maintains right to consult a lawyer and request a hearing
- Content of laws vary from state to state. Most states limit to 48 to 72 hours. Most permit commitment on one or more of the following three grounds
  - Dangerousness to self or others
  - Mentally ill and in need of treatment
  - Unable to provide for own basic needs

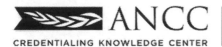
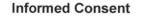
Informed Consent

454

- Person must be mentally competent and 18 or older (legal age of consent).
- For treatment, patient must be informed of and be able to understand:
  - Diagnosis,
  - Nature and purpose of proposed treatment,
  - Risks and consequences of proposed treatment,
  - Feasible alternative treatments,
  - Prognosis if treatment is not given,
  - Level of probability that treatment will be successful if patient complies with it, and
  - Free choice regarding treatment.
- Exception: Emergency risks to life or health that cannot wait.

Parent-Guardian Consent

455

- Necessary to provide medical or mental health care to minors (under age 18)
  - Minors must give written assent when participating in research studies.
- Exceptions: Court determined emancipated minor such as
  - Minor living separate and apart from parents or guardian who is managing his or her own financial affairs
  - Minor who is married or who has borne a child or served in the military
  - Parens patriae: The state acts a surrogate parent

Competence and Incompetence

456

- Competence
  - The ability to understand information provided, reason logically through to a decision, understand consequences, and clearly able to make a choice.
- Competency evaluations are recommended when the
  - Person has a mental disorder,
  - Disorder causes a defect in judgment, or a
  - Defect makes the person incapable of handling personal affairs.
- Incompetence
  - A legal term without a precise medical meaning.
  - Ruling requires the appointment of a legal guardian.

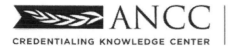
Review Question

457

- The nurse manager of a child and adolescent unit plans a study investigating the effects of music therapy on adolescent aggression on the inpatient unit. What is the primary responsibility of the nurse manager as it pertains to the tenets of National Commission for the Protection of Human Subjects of Biomedical and Behavioral Research?
- Assure that the Medical Director, Nurse Supervisor and IRB are involved.
- Obtain consent from the parents or guardians of the children and adolescents.
- Get assent from the adolescent participants.
- Do no harm or have a plan in place if potential for harm exists.

© 2014 American Nurses Credentialing Center

CATEGORY III C: LEADERSHIP

© 2014 American Nurses Credentialing Center

007: Nurse-Patient Relationships, Professional Development, & Leadership (Part 2)

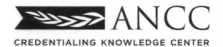
007: Learning Objectives   460

1. Identify RN roles that demonstrate leadership and professional accountability.
2. Discuss the importance of contributing to quality improvement in health systems.

© 2014 American Nurses Credentialing Center

Leadership and Management: Professional Performance Standard 15   461

- Leadership
  - The use of one's skills to direct and influence others to perform to the best of their ability.
  - Interpersonal process between leader and followers.
    - Transactional: Maintains the status quo.
    - Transformational: Changes the work culture.
- Management
  - Handles day-to-day operations of a work group to achieve a desired outcome.
    - Planning, staffing, organizing, direction, controlling, or decision making.
  - Effective managers may become leaders.

© 2014 American Nurses Credentialing Center

Good Leader Attributes and Behaviors   462

- Open-minded
- Consistent
- Responsible
- Strong character
- Ability to teach
- Excellent problem solver
- Excellent clinical skills
- Good sense of humor
- Active listener
- Sensitive

- Objective
- Flexible
- Decisive
- Calm
- Assertive
- Articulate
- Fair
- Organized Considerate
- Tactful
- Good role model

Conveys mutual trust, respect, warmth, rapport among staff; organizes and defines work to be accomplished; establishes well-defined work patterns and channels of communication.

© 2014 American Nurses Credentialing Center

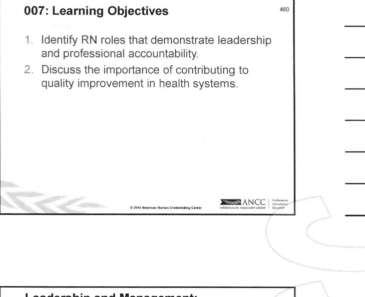

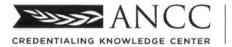
Leadership Styles

463

- Autocratic
  - Leader retains authority, makes decisions, establishes one-way communication with the work group (effective in crisis situations).
- Democratic
  - Leader focuses on teamwork and workgroup participation in decision-making (effective with mature staff).
- Laissez-faire
  - Leader gives up control with free-run or permissive style (effective with highly motivated staff).
- Transformational
  - Leader changes the work culture.
- Situational
  - Situation-dependent; is flexible (leader gradually gives more authority to staff).

© 2014 American Nurses Credentialing Center

Leadership Behaviors

464

- Directing: More important with new staff.

- Coaching: Good with staff who are more experienced but still need some guidance.

- Supporting: Assists staff in problem solving.

- Delegating: Transfers responsibility to staff while retaining accountability, and promotes staff development.

© 2014 American Nurses Credentialing Center

Effective Leadership and Management

465

- Collaboration evident

- Effective communication evident
  - Is specific about what is to be done, how it is to be done, and when it is to be completed.

- Clinical competence evident

© 2014 American Nurses Credentialing Center

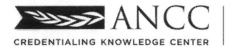
Effective Leadership and Management

466

- Organizational skills/time management
  - Staffing: Chooses the management structure, coordinating people, time, task assignments.
  - Recruiting: Hiring, training, scheduling, ongoing staff development.
  - Planning: Defining goals, objectives, policies, procedures, resource allocation.
  - Controlling: Conducting performance evaluations, analyzing financial activities, monitoring quality of care.
  - Supervising: Directing, guiding and influencing an individual's performance.

© 2014 American Nurses Credentialing Center

Effective Leadership and Management

467

- Conflict Resolution Principles
  - Identify conflict issues.
  - Know your own response to conflict.
  - Separate the problem from the people involved.
  - Stay focused on the issue and the underlying motivations of stakeholders.
  - Identify available options.
  - Mediate (settle differences).
  - Search for an outcome based on fair, objective criteria.

© 2014 American Nurses Credentialing Center

Effective Leadership and Management

468

- Conflict Resolution Styles
  - Avoidance: Differences not worth worrying about; avoid unpleasantness; avoid controversy.
  - Accommodation: Try to negotiate; soothes others feelings and preserve relationships.
  - Coerciveness: My way or highway.
  - Competition: Try to win; show logic/benefits of my position.
  - Compromise: I give, you give; seek intermediary position between two.
  - Collaboration: Try to work through; leans toward direct discussion.

© 2014 American Nurses Credentialing Center

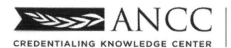
Effective Leadership and Management 469

- Conflict Resolution Strategies
  - Prepare for the encounter.
  - Manage own anxiety or anger.
  - Select an optimal time for the encounter.
  - Work on one issue at a time.
  - Make a request for behavioral change.
  - Keep in mind cultural differences.
  - Evaluate progress.

Professional Practice Evaluation: Standard 9 470

- Trending for the Future
  - To Err is Human: Institute of Medicine (IOM) publication.
    - Promoting safe and supportive working environments:
      - Transformational leadership.
      - Evidence-based management.
      - Maximize workforce capability.
      - Redesign work to detect and prevent errors.
      - Create and sustain a culture of safety.
  - Future of Nursing: ANA and IOM collaboration pub.
    - Nursing Residency Programs: Transition to Practice.
    - BSN, DNP degree requirements: 80% by 2020.

Supportive Work Environment 471

- Shared Governance structures
- Empathic
- Good leaders and managers
- Give clear directions
- Clear lines of authority
- Shows respect for individual differences
- Openly communicates about problems
- Displays positive approach to resolving impasses
- Talents and skills of others are genuinely recognized and celebrated

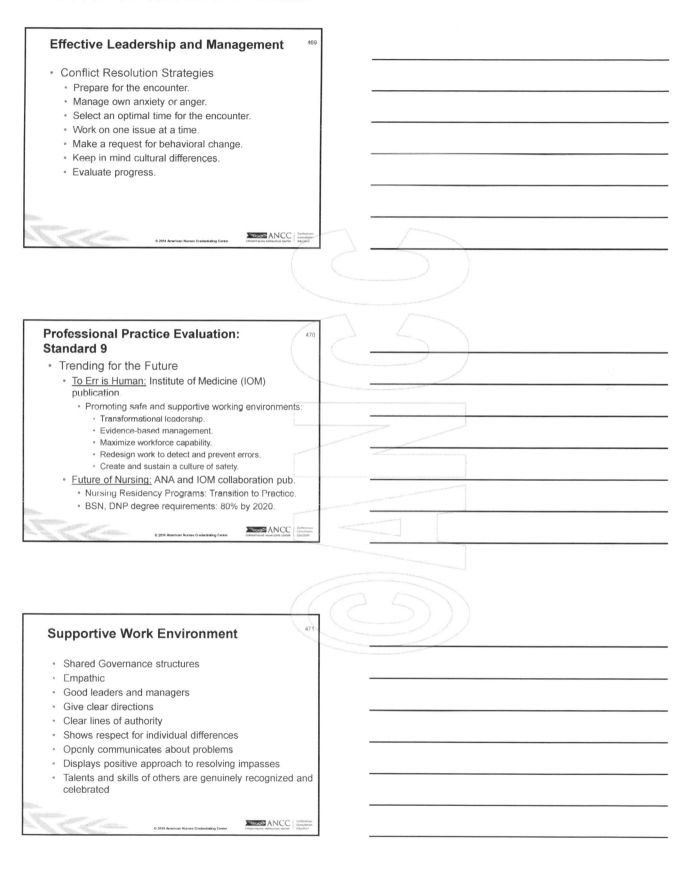

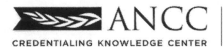
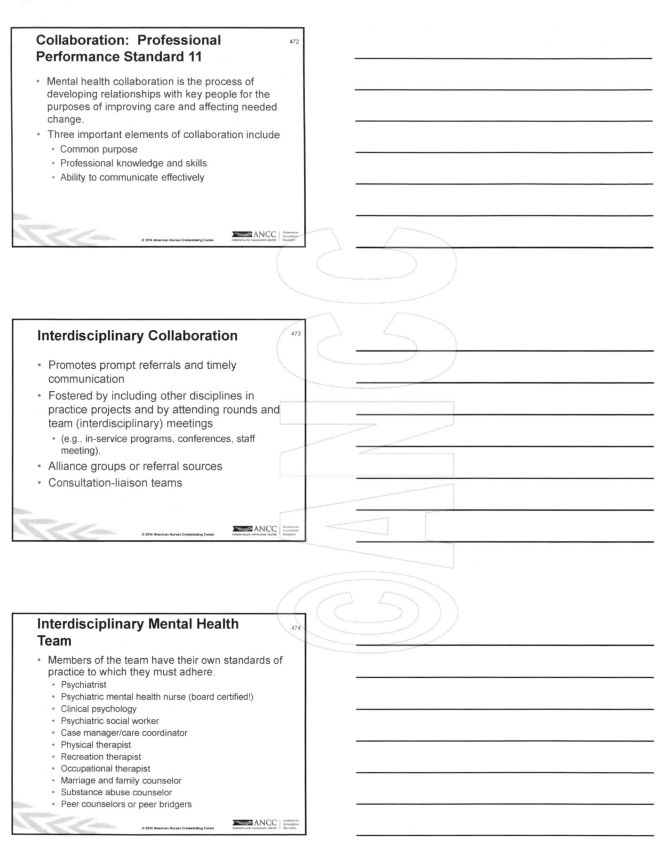

Collaboration: Professional Performance Standard 11

472

- Mental health collaboration is the process of developing relationships with key people for the purposes of improving care and affecting needed change.
- Three important elements of collaboration include
  - Common purpose
  - Professional knowledge and skills
  - Ability to communicate effectively

© 2014 American Nurses Credentialing Center

Interdisciplinary Collaboration

473

- Promotes prompt referrals and timely communication
- Fostered by including other disciplines in practice projects and by attending rounds and team (interdisciplinary) meetings
  - (e.g., in-service programs, conferences, staff meeting).
- Alliance groups or referral sources
- Consultation-liaison teams

© 2014 American Nurses Credentialing Center

Interdisciplinary Mental Health Team

474

- Members of the team have their own standards of practice to which they must adhere.
  - Psychiatrist
  - Psychiatric mental health nurse (board certified!)
  - Clinical psychology
  - Psychiatric social worker
  - Case manager/care coordinator
  - Physical therapist
  - Recreation therapist
  - Occupational therapist
  - Marriage and family counselor
  - Substance abuse counselor
  - Peer counselors or peer bridgers

© 2014 American Nurses Credentialing Center

Collaboration: Delegation Process

475

Delegator:

* Act of delegation.
* Supervises the delegated task.
* Assesses the task accomplishments.
* Intervenes or employs corrective actions to ensure quality care.
* Evaluates.

Delegatee:

* Accountable for own actions.
* Ensures the activity is within scope of practice and level of knowledge/competence.
* Effectively communicates with delegator.
* Completes assigned tasks.

© 2014 American Nurses Credentialing Center

Guidelines for Delegation

476

* State Nurse Practice Acts, institutional procedures, state laws.
* Job descriptions and competencies of delegatee.
* Complexity of the clinical situation.
* Professional Standards of Nursing Practice.
  * Only nursing tasks, not nursing practice can be delegated.
* Must transfer responsibility to those individuals with:
  * Appropriate skill
  * Sufficient knowledge and judgment
  * Within the person's scope of practice

© 2014 American Nurses Credentialing Center

Five Rights of Delegation

477

1. Right task
2. Right circumstances:
   * Tasks that do not require independent nursing judgment.
3. Right person
4. Right direction and communication:
   * Clear explanation, expected outcomes, reporting process.
5. Right supervision and evaluation

© 2014 American Nurses Credentialing Center

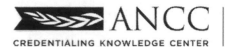
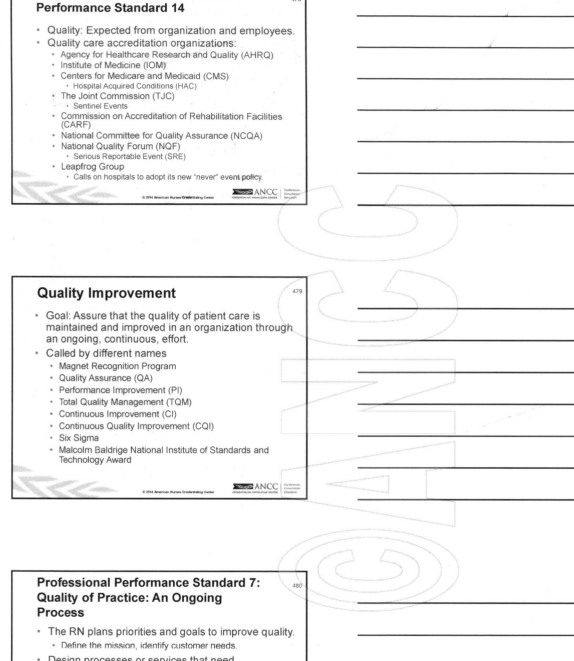

Resource Utilization: Professional Performance Standard 14   478

- Quality: Expected from organization and employees.
- Quality care accreditation organizations:
  - Agency for Healthcare Research and Quality (AHRQ)
  - Institute of Medicine (IOM)
  - Centers for Medicare and Medicaid (CMS)
    - Hospital Acquired Conditions (HAC)
  - The Joint Commission (TJC)
    - Sentinel Events
  - Commission on Accreditation of Rehabilitation Facilities (CARF)
  - National Committee for Quality Assurance (NCQA)
  - National Quality Forum (NQF)
    - Serious Reportable Event (SRE)
  - Leapfrog Group
    - Calls on hospitals to adopt its new "never" event policy.

© 2014 American Nurses Credentialing Center   ANCC

Quality Improvement   479

- Goal: Assure that the quality of patient care is maintained and improved in an organization through an ongoing, continuous, effort.
- Called by different names
  - Magnet Recognition Program
  - Quality Assurance (QA)
  - Performance Improvement (PI)
  - Total Quality Management (TQM)
  - Continuous Improvement (CI)
  - Continuous Quality Improvement (CQI)
  - Six Sigma
  - Malcolm Baldrige National Institute of Standards and Technology Award

© 2014 American Nurses Credentialing Center   ANCC

Professional Performance Standard 7: Quality of Practice: An Ongoing Process   480

- The RN plans priorities and goals to improve quality.
  - Define the mission, identify customer needs.
- Design processes or services that need improvement.
  - Describe current processes, localize problems, identify data that are needed.
  - Problems can be identified by sentinel events, incident reports, or chart audits.
- Root Cause Analysis: Identify root causes of problems.
  - Generate solutions to root causes and develop pilot (test) study.

© 2014 American Nurses Credentialing Center   ANCC

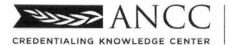
Quality of Practice: An Ongoing Process

481

- Measure performance
  - Test the pilot or collect data.
  - Outcome measures may include: Medication errors, functional outcomes, patient satisfaction, intervention times, and costs per capita.
- Analyze data
  - Evaluate the pilot; compare with baseline data.
- Improve practice
  - Standardize the new process or repeat; disseminate results.

© 2014 American Nurses Credentialing Center

Quality Components

482

- Professional standards
  - Authoritative statements that describe responsibilities for which nurses are held accountable.
  - An organization's interpretation of professional's competency.
  - Measured through professional outcomes and evaluations.
- Care guidelines
  - Systematically developed (evidence-based) statements to assist in determining appropriate care.
  - Include procedures, care plans, protocols, and critical pathways.
  - Measured though patient outcomes.

© 2014 American Nurses Credentialing Center

Quality Control Planning

483

- Quality values/statement/mission
  - What are the expected outcomes of this product or service?
  - What are the patient's expectations?
- Quality improvement infrastructure
  - What criteria define quality?
  - Leadership, QI teams, meeting structure, staff involvement, communication, education, and expectations.
- Annual quality goals
  - Review yearly goals and performance appraisals.
  - How will you know if expectations have been achieved?

© 2014 American Nurses Credentialing Center

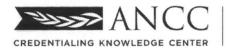
Quality Framework

484

The Joint Commission and The National Committee for Quality Assurance provides accreditation to organizations who maintain safety and quality of care. Organizations demonstrate this by:
1. Mission, Vision, and Value statements
2. Professional Standards
3. Care Guidelines

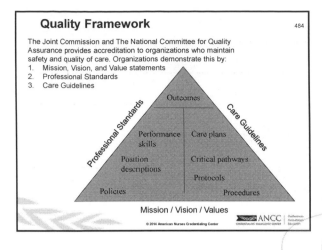

Leader Roles in QI

485

- Conveys importance and relevance of QI.
- Organizes educational activities to promote quality.
- Motivates and recognizes staff for their QI efforts.
- Institutionalizes quality improvement.
- Commits monies, time, and sufficient expertise.
- Provides feedback in the form of data (metrics) to demonstrate program successes and improve performance.
- Commit resources to support QI program.
- Act as a clinical champion, keeping the team on track.

Barriers to QI Success

486

- Lack of system support
- Lack of financial or time resources
- Conflicting organizational goals
- Insufficient expertise
- Lack of data feedback
- Information overload
- Lack of understanding regarding purpose

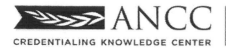

CATEGORY IV: PATIENT
EDUCATION AND POPULATION
HEALTH

© 2014 American Nurses Credentialing Center

CATEGORY IV A: PATIENT
EDUCATION

© 2014 American Nurses Credentialing Center

**008: Patient Education; Population
Health; Exam Preparation Resources**

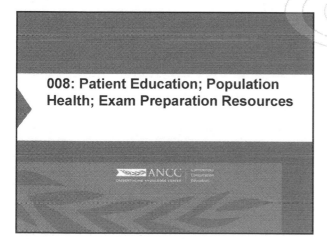

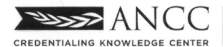
Session 008: Learning Objectives

490

1. Identify appropriate strategies for teaching-learning success in patient education as it relates to population health.
2. Identify counseling and other individual and group psychoeducational approaches that support patient-centered, family mental health.
3. Discuss the roles of the RN in advocating for the psychiatric mental health patient population, including eliminating stigma, discrimination, and criminalization.

© 2014 American Nurses Credentialing Center

Health Teaching and Health Promotion: Practice Standard 5B

491

* The professional RN provides teaching in health promotion and wellness behaviors incorporating principles of levels of prevention.
* Process of patient education
  * Assessment of need, readiness, ability and motivation to learn.
  * Assessment of developmental stage and appropriate teaching-learning strategies.
  * Assessment of other barriers to educational access or success.
  * Importance of developing educational objectives.
  * Teaching-learning engagement.
  * Evaluation and re-teaching if necessary.

© 2014 American Nurses Credentialing Center

Nurse and Patient: Mutual Teach and Learn

492

* Goal: Development of an individualized plan of care with the patient that facilitates knowledge, and engagement in self-management of illness, promotion of personal health and wellness, management of medications, creation of a crisis safety plan, and relapse prevention support.
* Cognitive, mental, and physical development affects learner ability to learn, comprehend, and apply knowledge.
* Therapeutic culturally sensitive communication skills are essential for optimal transfer and acceptance of learned material.

© 2014 American Nurses Credentialing Center

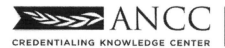

Health Promotion

493

- Pender describes "cues to action" as health perceptions and beliefs about one's susceptibility, disease severity, consequences, or effectiveness of interventions.
- Promoting health can
  - Reduce anxiety, stress, pain, and suffering
  - Enable attainment of life goals
  - Reduce health care costs
- Passive strategies
  - Benefits gained without personal action (e.g., no smoking policies)
- Active strategies
  - Health education programs (e.g., weight reduction, smoking cessation classes)

Health Promotion and Wellness Standards

494

- Self-care promotion
  - Psycho-education groups (develop skills; manage stress; safety plan; medication adherence)
  - Encourage patient to verbalize feelings
  - Encourage positive self-talk
  - Enforce beneficial activities such as good nutrition, added sleep, exercise, and so on
- Health promotion and health maintenance
  - Parenting skills classes for teenage mothers
  - Reminiscence groups for elders in nursing homes.
  - Teach process of self-reward
  - Reinforce past and new coping skills
  - Discourage negative thinking

Functional Health Patterns: Womb to Tomb

405

Wellness promotion	Well-being promotion
"I feel good," or "I participate in good choices," or "I understand"	"I am OK," or "I am good enough" or "I know and I believe"
• Health perception	• Self-perception
• Health management	• Self-concept
• Nutrition-metabolism	• Roles-relationships
• Elimination	• Sexuality-reproduction
• Activity-exercise	• Coping-stress tolerance
• Sleep-rest	• Value-beliefs
	• Cognition-perceptions

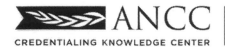
Health Literacy

496

* The degree to which individuals have the capacity to obtain, process, and understand basic health information and services needed to make appropriate health decisions and follow instructions for treatment (Institute of Medicine).

© 2014 American Nurses Credentialing Center

Assess Need, Readiness, Ability to Learn

497

* Consider Maslow's Hierarchy of Needs Theory
  * Physiologic and survival, safety and security, love and belonging, self-esteem, self-actualization, and self-transcendence
* Consider readiness
  * Life experiences, complexity of task, language, culture, values, beliefs, level of anxiety, social support, the environment, the feedback, personal health status

* Consider ability
  * Developmental level; cognitive abilities
* Question
  * What do you know about your illness and treatment?
  * How do you cope with the symptoms?
  * What concerns you the most right now?

© 2014 American Nurses Credentialing Center

Assessment of Health Beliefs

498

* Perceptions and beliefs influence the likelihood that a person will take action regarding
  * Susceptibility to illness
  * Seriousness of the illness
  * Benefits and barriers of taking action
* Preventive actions include
  * Lifestyle changes
  * Increased adherence to medical therapies
  * Seek medical advice or treatment when appropriate

© 2014 American Nurses Credentialing Center

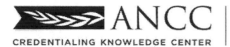
Factors That Influence Health Beliefs

499

- Internal (internal locus of control)
  - Developmental stage
  - Intellectual background
  - Perception of functioning
  - Emotional factors
  - Spiritual factors
- External (external locus of control)
  - Family practices
  - Socioeconomic factors
  - Cultural background

© 2014 American Nurses Credentialing Center

Assessment of Motivation

500

- Health Belief Model
  - Individuals unlikely to take health actions unless they:
    - Believe they are susceptible to the ill-health condition in question,
    - Believe the condition would seriously affect their lives if they should contract it,
    - Believe that benefits of action outweigh barriers to action, and
    - Believe they are confident that they can perform the action (definition of self-efficacy).

© 2014 American Nurses Credentialing Center

Assessing Motivation to Change: Five Stages of Change Model

501

- Also called Transtheoretical Model of Behavior Change (Prochaska & DiClemente,1986)
1. Precontemplation: No intention to change.
   - Raise doubt; increase perception of risks and problems with current behavior, "I never thought about quitting smoking."
2. Contemplation: Awareness that a problem exists.
   - Tip the balance; evoke a reason to change; Consider risk of not changing, "I have thought of quitting, maybe someday."
3. Preparation: Ready for change.
   - Help to determine best course of action to take in seeking change, "I will put a quit date on my calendar."
4. Action: Taking overt steps.
   - Help to take steps toward change, "I will toss my ashtrays and lighters."
5. Maintenance: Work to prevent relapse.
   - Help to identify and use strategies to prevent relapse, "I failed."

© 2014 American Nurses Credentialing Center

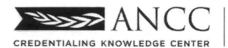

Change: Dynamics and Barriers 502

Dynamics	Barriers

• Change
   • Essential for adaptation and growth
• Change agent
   • Works to bring about change
• Driving forces
   • Behaviors facilitating change
• Restraining forces
   • Behaviors impeding change
	• Desire to maintain the status quo
	• Change is threatening
	• Negative past experiences
	• Lack of support
	• Unrealistic solutions
	• Lack of understanding

© 2014 American Nurses Credentialing Center

_____

_____

_____

_____

_____

_____

Change: Process and Strategies 503

Process	Strategies

• Assessment
   • Identify problems
   • Collect/analyze data
• Planning
   • Who, how, when to change
• Implementation
   • Individual and group methods
• Evaluation
   • Monitor effectiveness
	• Unfreeze existing equilibrium
	   • Motivate for change
	   • Build trust/recognition for change
	   • Identify problems/solutions
	• Move to new equilibrium level
	   • Agree that status quo not beneficial
	   • Gain acceptance
	• Refreeze at new equilibrium level
	   • Stabilize and reinforce new behavior patterns

© 2014 American Nurses Credentialing Center

_____

_____

_____

_____

Motivational Interviewing 504

- Derived from Stages of Change Theory (Miller & Rollnick, 1991)
  - Counseling style that uses form of communication that strengthens personal motivation to change.
  - Addresses problem of ambivalence about change by paying attention to the language of change.
  - Technique fosters an atmosphere of acceptance and compassion.

© 2014 American Nurses Credentialing Center

_____

_____

_____

_____

_____

_____

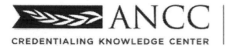
Planning Health Teaching: Womb to Tomb

505

- Educational Objectives:
  - A statement of goals and objectives that constitute a plan for instruction.
  - Requires the use of terms with precise meanings, a statement of both a behavior and a content, such that the outcome can be evaluated.
  - Three domains for objectives
    - Cognitive (content)
    - Affective (feeling)
    - Psychomotor (practice/doing)
- Patient population concepts:
  - Pedagogy: Art and science of educating children.
  - Androgogy: Art and science of educating adults.

© 2014 American Nurses Credentialing Center

Developmental Stage and Teaching Strategies

506

- Infant/Toddler (Birth to 3 years)
  - Sensorimotor
  - Trust vs. mistrust
  - Autonomy vs. shame
- Teaching Strategies
  - Repetition and imitation
  - Stimulate all senses
  - Provide physical safety and emotional security
  - Play and object manipulation

- Preschooler (3 to 6 years)
  - Preoperational
  - Initiative vs. guilt
- Teaching Strategies
  - Repetition
  - Object manipulation and technology
  - Reassurance
  - Simple explanations
  - Positive reinforcement
  - Simple drawings and stories
  - Play therapy

© 2014 American Nurses Credentialing Center

Developmental Stage and Teaching Strategies

507

School-Aged (6 to 12 years)
- Concrete operations
- Industry vs. inferiority
- Teaching strategies
  - Encourage independence and active participation.
  - Use logical explanation.
  - Use analogies to make invisible processes real.
  - Relate to other experiences.
  - Play and group activities
  - Drawings, models, dolls, painting, audio, video, technology.

Adolescence (12 to 18 years)
- Formal operations
- Identity vs. role confusion
- Teaching strategies
  - Establish trust, authenticity
  - Include in plan of care.
  - Use peers for support.
  - Negotiate changes.
  - Make information meaningful.
  - Audiovisuals, role-play, group work, reading materials, technology.

© 2014 American Nurses Credentialing Center

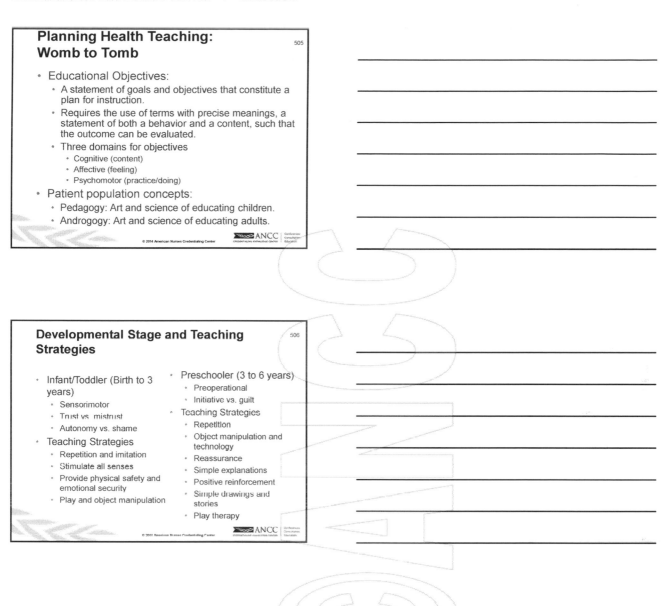

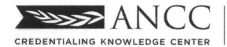
Developmental Stage and Teaching Strategies

508

Young Adulthood (18 to 40 years)
- Formal operations
- Intimacy vs. isolation
- Teaching strategies
  - Active participation.
  - Set own pace, self-directed.
  - Draw on meaningful experiences.
  - Apply new knowledge through role-playing and hands-on practice; technology.

Middle-Aged Adulthood (40 to 65 years)
- Formal operations
- Generativity vs. self-absorption and stagnation
- Teaching strategies
  - Focus on maintaining independence and reestablishing normal life patterns.
  - Provide information to coincide with life concerns and problems.
  - Telehealth; technology.

© 2014 American Nurses Credentialing Center

Developmental Stage and Teaching Strategies

509

- Elder Adults
- Cognitive and psychosocial stages
  - Formal operations
  - Ego integrity vs. despair
- Teaching strategies
  - Use concrete examples; build on past life experiences
  - Make information relevant and meaningful
  - Present one concept at a time; allow time for processing
  - Repetition and reinforcement
  - Keep explanations brief; use analogies to illustrate abstract info
  - Speak slowly, distinctly; minimize distractions
  - Use large letters and well-spaced print with simple, clear presentation; avoid written exams

© 2014 American Nurses Credentialing Center

Patient Education: Promote Safe Sex

510

- Use protection at each encounter.
- Practice monogamous relationships.
- Know one's sexual partner.
- Discuss sexual and drug-use history with partner.
- Don't let drugs/alcohol influence decisions about using protection.
- Get tested.
- Get immunized.

© 2014 American Nurses Credentialing Center

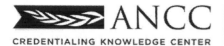
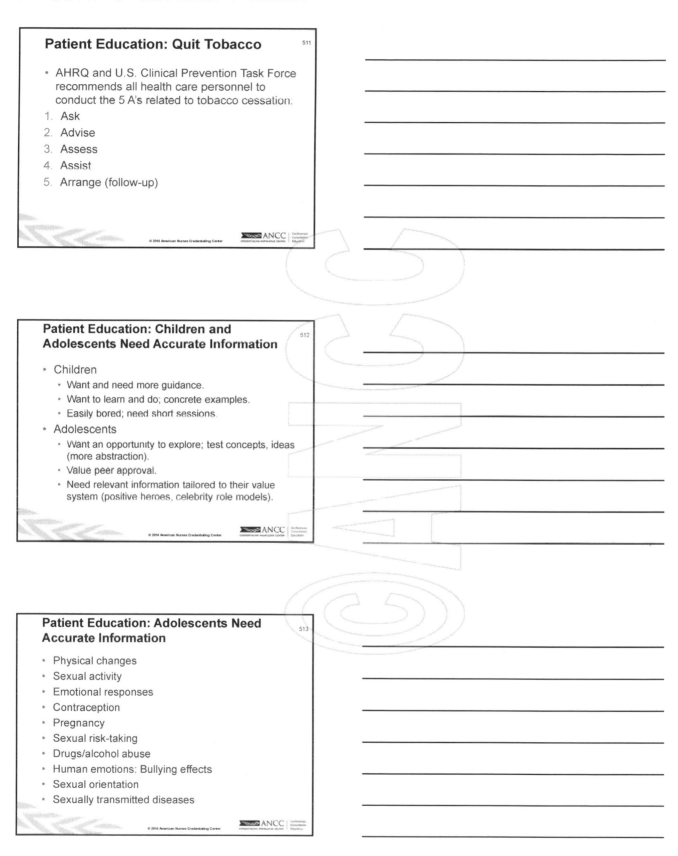

Patient Education: Quit Tobacco 511

- AHRQ and U.S. Clinical Prevention Task Force recommends all health care personnel to conduct the 5 A's related to tobacco cessation.
1. Ask
2. Advise
3. Assess
4. Assist
5. Arrange (follow-up)

© 2014 American Nurses Credentialing Center

Patient Education: Children and Adolescents Need Accurate Information 512

- Children
  - Want and need more guidance.
  - Want to learn and do; concrete examples.
  - Easily bored; need short sessions.
- Adolescents
  - Want an opportunity to explore; test concepts, ideas (more abstraction).
  - Value peer approval.
  - Need relevant information tailored to their value system (positive heroes, celebrity role models).

© 2014 American Nurses Credentialing Center

Patient Education: Adolescents Need Accurate Information 513

- Physical changes
- Sexual activity
- Emotional responses
- Contraception
- Pregnancy
- Sexual risk-taking
- Drugs/alcohol abuse
- Human emotions: Bullying effects
- Sexual orientation
- Sexually transmitted diseases

© 2014 American Nurses Credentialing Center

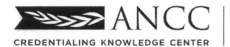
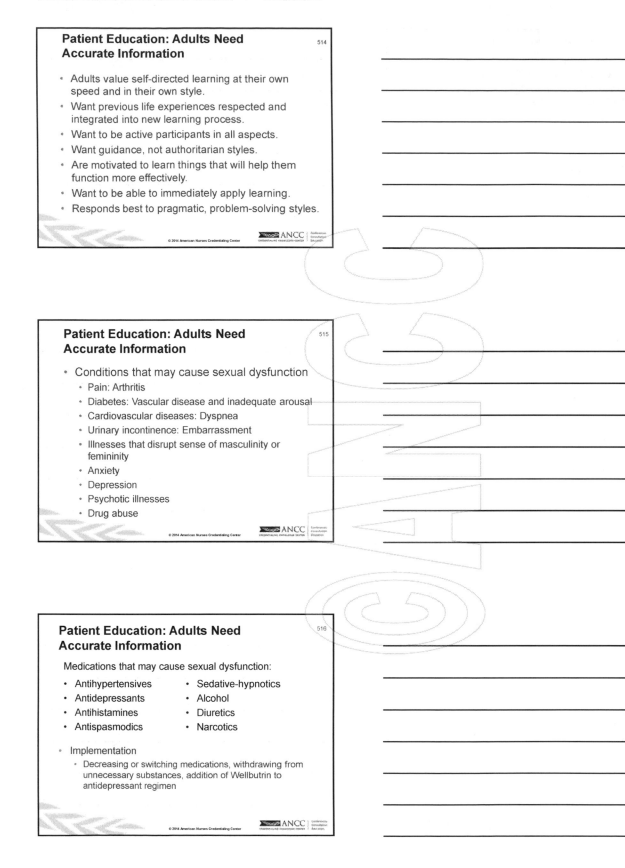

Patient Education: Adults Need Accurate Information   514

- Adults value self-directed learning at their own speed and in their own style.
- Want previous life experiences respected and integrated into new learning process.
- Want to be active participants in all aspects.
- Want guidance, not authoritarian styles.
- Are motivated to learn things that will help them function more effectively.
- Want to be able to immediately apply learning.
- Responds best to pragmatic, problem-solving styles.

Patient Education: Adults Need Accurate Information   515

- Conditions that may cause sexual dysfunction
  - Pain: Arthritis
  - Diabetes: Vascular disease and inadequate arousal
  - Cardiovascular diseases: Dyspnea
  - Urinary incontinence: Embarrassment
  - Illnesses that disrupt sense of masculinity or femininity
  - Anxiety
  - Depression
  - Psychotic illnesses
  - Drug abuse

Patient Education: Adults Need Accurate Information   516

Medications that may cause sexual dysfunction:

- Antihypertensives
- Antidepressants
- Antihistamines
- Antispasmodics
- Sedative-hypnotics
- Alcohol
- Diuretics
- Narcotics

- Implementation
  - Decreasing or switching medications, withdrawing from unnecessary substances, addition of Wellbutrin to antidepressant regimen

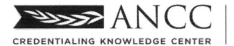
Patient Education: Elders Need Accurate Information

517

- Keep explanations brief but accurate.
- Speak slowly and distinctly.
- Minimize distractions.
- Use concrete examples.
- Build on past life experiences.
- Make information relevant and meaningful.
- Present one concept at a time.
- Allow time for processing.
- Repeat and reinforce.

© 2014 American Nurses Credentialing Center

Health Teaching and Health Promotion: Summary

518

- Match teaching to developmental stage, learning style, and learning needs. Active, interactive methods result in greater behavioral change.
- Learner's reaction: Learning may be most effective when the teacher uses a variety of teaching approaches. Structure learning choices to develop self-directed learning skills.
- Acquisition of knowledge/skills. Modifies attitudes/perceptions.
- Change in behavior. Benefits to patients.
- Change in organizational practice.

© 2014 American Nurses Credentialing Center

Three Levels of Prevention

519

1. Primary prevention: Aims to remove potential risks.
   - Health promotion activities in the absence of disease
2. Secondary prevention: Early detection of disease with the aim of reversing or halting its progress.
   - Health screenings
3. Tertiary prevention: Prevent deterioration and complications when disease or disability is already established.
   - Rehabilitation treatment; curative

© 2014 American Nurses Credentialing Center

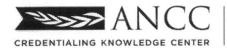
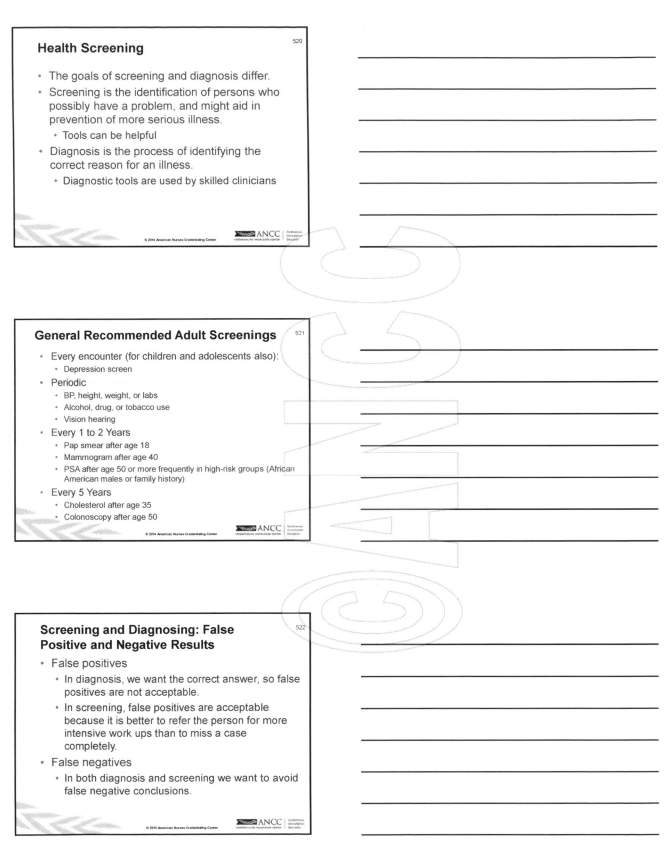

Health Screening

520

- The goals of screening and diagnosis differ.
- Screening is the identification of persons who possibly have a problem, and might aid in prevention of more serious illness.
  - Tools can be helpful
- Diagnosis is the process of identifying the correct reason for an illness.
  - Diagnostic tools are used by skilled clinicians

General Recommended Adult Screenings

521

- Every encounter (for children and adolescents also):
  - Depression screen
- Periodic
  - BP, height, weight, or labs
  - Alcohol, drug, or tobacco use
  - Vision hearing
- Every 1 to 2 Years
  - Pap smear after age 18
  - Mammogram after age 40
  - PSA after age 50 or more frequently in high-risk groups (African American males or family history)
- Every 5 Years
  - Cholesterol after age 35
  - Colonoscopy after age 50

Screening and Diagnosing: False Positive and Negative Results

522

- False positives
  - In diagnosis, we want the correct answer, so false positives are not acceptable.
  - In screening, false positives are acceptable because it is better to refer the person for more intensive work ups than to miss a case completely.
- False negatives
  - In both diagnosis and screening we want to avoid false negative conclusions.

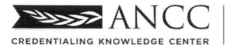
CAGE: Screening for Alcohol (or other drug) Problems

523

Four question screening assessment:

1. Have you ever felt the need to Cut down on your drinking?
2. Have you ever felt Annoyed by criticism of drinking?
3. Have you ever felt Guilty about drinking?
4. Have you ever taken a drink first thing in the morning (Eye-opener) to steady your nerves or get rid of a hangover?
   - Score 2 or more "yes" = suggestive for alcohol disorder; treatment decision, documentation of plan or referral.
   - Score 1 "yes" = hazardous drinking.

© 2014 American Nurses Credentialing Center

Grief and Loss at End-of-Life

524

- Universal Stages of Death and Dying
  - Anticipation: Sometimes possible
  - Denial: "No, not me."
  - Anger: "Why me?"
  - Bargaining: "Yes me…BUT…"
  - Depression: "Yes, me (groan)"
  - Acceptance: "It will be OK."

Kubler-Ross, E. and Kessler, D. (2005). On grief and grieving

© 2014 American Nurses Credentialing Center

End-of-Life Anticipatory Planning

525

- Begin the emotional work before the actual loss.
- Reminisce; recall milestones.
- Inquire about spiritual/religious beliefs.
- Allow expressions of sadness.
- Assist in transition from hope for recovery to hope for a peaceful, dignified death.
- Alert school nurse or counselor to help children with loss or death in family.

© 2014 American Nurses Credentialing Center

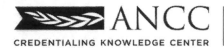
End-of-Life Care

526

- Nurse as advocate…
  - Often the caregiver that becomes aware of the need for a family meeting to discuss end-of-life care issues.
  - May facilitate family decision-making, palliative, or hospice care.
  - Encourages the family to develop Advanced Directives.
  - Pain management and comfort care support.

© 2014 American Nurses Credentialing Center

Psychiatric Advance Directives

527

- RN documentation allows a patient to:
  - Register refusal of certain psychiatric interventions, such as ECT and certain psychotropic medications.
  - Specify conditions under which these interventions are acceptable.
  - Appoint a trusted surrogate decision maker; a person authorized to give consent on the one's behalf.
  - Register willingness to participate in research studies.
  - Improve communication between the person and mental health team.
    http://www.myplanmylife.com/

© 2014 American Nurses Credentialing Center

Implementations: Death and Dying

528

- Communication strategies
  - Identify patient goals and expectations of care and treatment.
  - Avoid euphemisms for words like death and dying.
  - Be specific when using words such as "hope" and "better."
  - Listen to and honor preferences, values, and cultural beliefs.

© 2014 American Nurses Credentialing Center

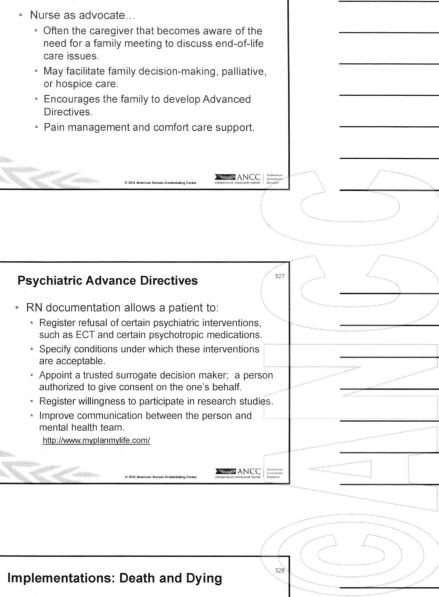

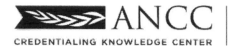
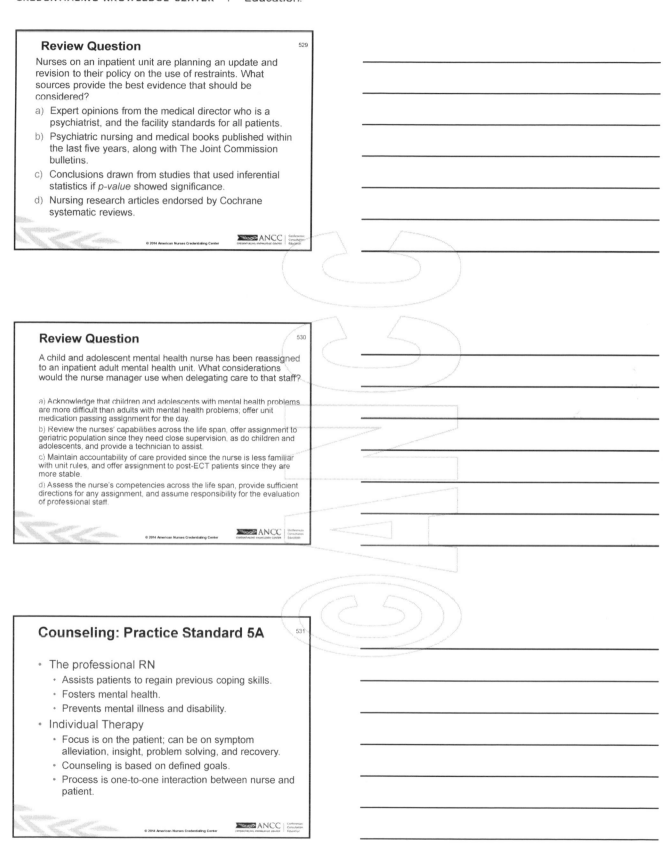

Review Question 529

Nurses on an inpatient unit are planning an update and revision to their policy on the use of restraints. What sources provide the best evidence that should be considered?

a) Expert opinions from the medical director who is a psychiatrist, and the facility standards for all patients.

b) Psychiatric nursing and medical books published within the last five years, along with The Joint Commission bulletins.

c) Conclusions drawn from studies that used inferential statistics if *p-value* showed significance.

d) Nursing research articles endorsed by Cochrane systematic reviews.

Review Question 530

A child and adolescent mental health nurse has been reassigned to an inpatient adult mental health unit. What considerations would the nurse manager use when delegating care to that staff?

a) Acknowledge that children and adolescents with mental health problems are more difficult than adults with mental health problems; offer unit medication passing assignment for the day.

b) Review the nurses' capabilities across the life span, offer assignment to geriatric population since they need close supervision, as do children and adolescents, and provide a technician to assist.

c) Maintain accountability of care provided since the nurse is less familiar with unit rules, and offer assignment to post-ECT patients since they are more stable.

d) Assess the nurse's competencies across the life span, provide sufficient directions for any assignment, and assume responsibility for the evaluation of professional staff.

Counseling: Practice Standard 5A 531

* The professional RN
    * Assists patients to regain previous coping skills.
    * Fosters mental health.
    * Prevents mental illness and disability.
* Individual Therapy
    * Focus is on the patient; can be on symptom alleviation, insight, problem solving, and recovery.
    * Counseling is based on defined goals.
    * Process is one-to-one interaction between nurse and patient.

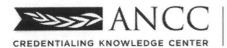

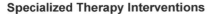

Specialized Therapy Interventions 532

- Preventative Psychiatry (Caplan)
- Cognitive-Behavioral Therapy (Beck; Ellis)
- Dialectical Behavioral Therapy (Lineham)
- Psychoanalysis (Freud)
- Behavior Modification (Skinner; Bandura)
- Group Therapy (Yalom; Tuckman)
- Family Therapy (Minuchin; Bowen; Haley and Madanes)
- Multimodal Therapy
- Therapeutic Communities (Jones)
- Eye Movement Desensitization and Reprocessing (Shapiro): Effective treating PTSD

© 2014 American Nurses Credentialing Center

Cognitive Behavioral Therapy (CBT) 533

- Cognitive theory
  - Distortions lead to behavioral and emotional problems.
  - Emphasis is on changing maladaptive thinking, perceptions, and attitudes
- CBT approaches
  - Identification of distressing emotions, related thought content, irrational beliefs, and schemas
  - Homework assignments, in the form of self-monitoring logs, or positive self-talk expected
  - Techniques: Practice and role playing

© 2014 American Nurses Credentialing Center

Cognitive Therapy: Goals and Processes 534

- Goals
  - Modify inaccurate and dysfunctional thinking.
  - Correct faulty perceptions.
  - Learn to differentiate own thoughts with events that are reality-based.
  - Acquire insight (long-term goal) about connection between thinking and behavior/feeling.
- Processes
  - Socratic dialogue to test beliefs: "What evidence do you have that ...?"
  - Review activity records to gather and test assumptions.
  - Help patient form alternative interpretations.

© 2014 American Nurses Credentialing Center

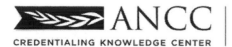
Behavioral Therapy

535

- Behavioral theorists
  - BF Skinner: Positive and Negative Reinforcement.
  - Albert Bandura: Social Learning Theory; Self-Efficacy.
    - Perception of one's ability to perform successfully and belief that action leads to desired outcome. "How confident...?"
- Behavioral theory
  - All behavior is learned, therefore, can be unlearned (learned helplessness).
- Behavioral therapy approaches
  - Deal with patient's present problems.
  - Is an action-oriented, short-term approach.
  - Patient monitors own behaviors during and outside of therapy sessions (logs, diaries).
  - Emphasizes teaching self-management skills.

© 2014 American Nurses Credentialing Center

Behavioral Therapy

536

- Behavioral theory approaches
  - Behavior changes according to its immediate consequences; reinforcement strengthens behavior.
  - Learning is the development of insights or understandings that provide a potential guide for behavior.
  - Actions followed by good outcomes are likely to recur; actions followed by bad outcomes are less likely to occur.
  - Change the consequence and behavior likely to change.
  - Frequency of behaviors is influenced by antecedents and consequences.

© 2014 American Nurses Credentialing Center

Behavioral Therapy Concepts

537

- Positive Reinforcement: Increase with rewards.
- Negative Reinforcement: Increase by removing an aversive stimulus. "You will receive your medication via injection if you will not take it by mouth."
- Punishment: Reduce by administering an aversive stimulus or by removing a positive stimulus.
- Contingency Contracts: Specify behavior to change; rewards to earn; time frame.
- Token Economy: Earn tokens or stars when displaying appropriate behaviors.
- Extinction: Reduce by ignoring.

© 2014 American Nurses Credentialing Center

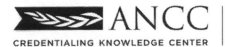
Behavior Modification Using Principles of Behavioral Therapy

538

- Reinforcement of positive response strategies
  - Privilege systems
  - Consistent limit setting
  - Modeling; shaping; discrimination
- Techniques
  - Directly observe behavior to establish a baseline
  - Define desired behavior as specifically as possible
  - Record the behavior and measuring its strength
  - Identify a meaningful reinforcer
  - Require performance of desired behavior to obtain the reinforcer
  - Vary the reinforcement schedule

ANCC
© 2014 American Nurses Credentialing Center

Behavioral Therapy: Systematic Desensitization

539

- Principles based on classical conditioning:
  - Pair an unconditioned response (relaxation) with a conditioned stimulus (feared event) to extinguish the unwanted behavior.
- Three steps: relaxation training, hierarchy construction, desensitization of stimulus:
  - Events or images are experienced hierarchically from least anxiety-provoking to most anxiety-provoking.
  - Patient is gradually desensitized to stimuli that produces undesired behavior.
- Useful in treating phobias, obsessions, compulsions, depression, and stuttering.

ANCC
© 2014 American Nurses Credentialing Center

Play Therapy with Children

540

- A dynamic process between the child and nurse (therapist) using play as the primary medium/implement.
  - Child explores at own pace the issues that may be affecting present life.
- Non-Directive
  - Child selects play materials and does not receive any specific suggestions from the therapist.
- Directive
  - Therapist selects and makes available play materials based on the child's age and the nature of the presenting problem and explicitly suggests to the child that he/she engage in a specific activity.

ANCC
© 2014 American Nurses Credentialing Center

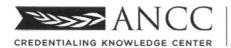
Play Therapy: Goals and Materials

541

- Goals
  - Catharsis and labeling of feelings
  - Corrective emotional experiences
  - Insight and working through
  - Exhibits adaptive problem solving and coping skills
  - Improved peer, school, home functioning
  - Developmental growth

- Materials/Implements
  - Drama, puppets, or storytelling
  - Art, sand, or clay
  - Dolls, games, or puzzles
  - Props
  - Family pictures
  - Music
  - Manipulatives
  - Books

© 2014 American Nurses Credentialing Center

Multimodal Therapy

542

- Theorist
  - Arnold Lazarus.
- Multimodal therapy
  - Addresses the seven dimensions of personality.
  - BASIC ID: **B**ehavior, **A**ffect, **S**ensation, **I**magery, **C**ognition and **I**nterpersonal relationships, and **D**rugs and biology.
- Multimodal therapy approaches
  - Must be multi-dimensional in examining each personality dimension to find the right therapy combination to address all seven dimensions.

© 2014 American Nurses Credentialing Center

CATEGORY IV B: POPULATION HEALTH

© 2014 American Nurses Credentialing Center

Group Work: Purposes

544

- Facilitates change when individual work meets impasse.

- Increases interpersonal learning and skill development.

- Is cost-effective: Several people benefit from intervention at once.

Group Principles, Facilitation, Development

545

- Principles of group therapy:
  - Members must have the capacity to engage in activities and communicate; can be heterogeneous or homogenous; can be closed or open formats.

Orientation ⟷	Forming
Transition ⟷	Storming
Cohesiveness ⟷	Norming
Working ⟷	Performing
Termination ⟷	Adjourning

Forming Stage (Orientation)

546

- Members
  - Risk-taking is low; tentative disclosure.
  - Major concerns: Inclusion, trust, and confidentiality.
  - Learning attitudinal behavioral expectations: Respect, acceptance, trust, and ways of responding.

- Nurse (as facilitator)
  - Establishes trust and rapport.
  - Helps mesh individual with group goals.
  - Provides structure and facilitate communication between members.

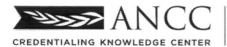

Conferences.
Consultation.
Education.

Storming Phase (Transition)

547

- Members
  - Increase conflict and struggle for control.
  - Expressions of "here and now" feelings.

- Nurse (as facilitator)
  - Recognize and express reactions.
  - Facilitates less defensive communication.
  - Keep to topic.
  - Inclusive to all.

© 2014 American Nurses Credentialing Center

Norming Phase (Cohesiveness)

548

- Members
  - Establish specific group norms.
  - Develop sense of cohesiveness.
  - Hold each other accountable.

- Nurse (as facilitator)
  - Helps members establish realistic group norms.
  - Reconciles norms with group goals.
  - Accepts diversity among group members.
  - Reinforces desired behaviors.

© 2014 American Nurses Credentialing Center

Performing Phase (Working)

549

- Members
  - Commit to group.
  - In-depth sharing and working through problems.
  - Working toward mutually set goals.
  - Hanging in there.
- Nurse (as facilitator)
  - Provides reinforcement.
  - Helps members connect themes.
  - Encourages members to practice new skills.
  - Supports risk-taking and constructive confrontation.
    - That is respectful, sensitive, direct, honest, and timely.

© 2014 American Nurses Credentialing Center

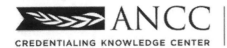

Adjourning Phase (Termination)

550

- Members
  - Express and deal with any final issues.

- Nurse (as facilitator)
  - Puts work into perspective; summarizes.
  - Reinforces transfer of learning into personal life.
  - Reinforces group accountability of confidentiality.
  - Deals with feelings about termination.
  - Expresses and deals with unfinished business.
  - Reinforces transferability of learning to patient lives.
  - Reminds of imminent termination.
  - Reinforces communication of final good-byes.

© 2014 American Nurses Credentialing Center

Irvin Yalom's 11 Curative Factors in Therapeutic Groups

551

1. Instillation of hope
   - Members at different levels of growth can gain hope from others that change is possible.
2. Universality
   - Discover that others have similar problems, thoughts, or feelings.
3. Altruism
   - Results from sharing oneself with another.
4. Increased development of socialization skills
   - Learn new social skills.
   - Correct maladaptive social behaviors.
5. Imitative behaviors
   - Increase skills by imitating behaviors of others.

© 2014 American Nurses Credentialing Center

Irvin Yalom's 11 Curative Factors in Therapeutic Groups (cont.)

552

6. Interpersonal learning
   - Interacting increases adaptive interpersonal relationships.
7. Group cohesiveness
   - Attraction to group and other members.
   - Promotes a sense of belonging.
8. Catharsis
   - Open expression of feeling previously unexpressed.
9. Existential factors
   - Enables member to deal with meaning of own existence.
10. Corrective refocusing
    - Re-experiences family conflict in the group (sibling and authority issues).
11. Imparting information

© 2014 American Nurses Credentialing Center

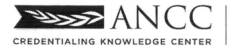
RN Facilitated Groups

553

- Psychoeducational
- Socialization
- Reality Orientation
- Reminiscence
- Therapeutic Activity
- Special Populations
- Medication Management
- Problem-Solving Training
- Relaxation-Based Treatments
- Communication Skills
- Assertive Training
- Modeling
- Support or Self-Help

© 2014 American Nurses Credentialing Center

Psychoeducational Groups

554

- Goals
  - Develop self-care skills, provide support, and/or learn about specific disorders
- Useful for the general population
  - Parenting skills
  - Stress management
- Useful for patients with physical or mental disorders
  - Medication
  - Coping with illnesses (cancer, heart disease, or schizophrenia)

© 2014 American Nurses Credentialing Center

Socialization and Social Skills Groups

555

- Goals
  - Develop basic skills of communication with others
  - Improve social skills
  - Increase social contacts
- Based on Social Cognitive Theory
  - Acquire information, develop values, attitudes, moral judgments, standards of behavior, and new behaviors by observing others
- Useful for withdrawn patients

© 2014 American Nurses Credentialing Center

Assertiveness Training

556

- Goals:
  - Learn to behave assertively in accord with self-integrity and sensitivity to others, such as "I" language.
  - Improve managing anger and other strong emotions.
  - Nurse teaches and models desired behaviors.
  - Initially rehearsed in the therapy environment.
  - Enacted on the outside.
- Useful in equipping persons with skills and attitudes to deal effectively with various interpersonal situations.

© 2014 American Nurses Credentialing Center

Special Population Groups

557

- Reality Orientation
  - Goals
    - Help patients maintain contact with environment.
    - Reduce confusion about person, place, and time.
    - Useful for confused, disoriented patients or populations.
- Reminiscence Groups
  - Goals
    - Review life experiences and significant events.
    - Improve socialization and self-esteem.
    - Useful for elders in ego integrity versus despair life stages.

© 2014 American Nurses Credentialing Center

Special Population Groups

558

- Self-Help Groups
  - Examples
    - Screening, Brief Intervention, and Referral to Treatment (SBIRT) in Primary Care is an evidence-based substance use initiative.
    - AA, Al-Anon, Chronic Pain Outreach, Overeaters Anonymous, Weight Watchers.
- Useful for persons and families who experience chronic illness, crises, or ill health of a family member.

© 2014 American Nurses Credentialing Center

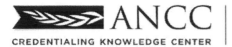

Special Population: Adolescents

559

- Characteristics that lend well to group techniques:
  - Strong need for identity to affirm self-image and peer acceptance is extremely important; behavioral standards are set by peer group.
  - Conflicts between dependence and independence, can be detected and addressed more easily by peers.
- Forming stage:
  - Begin with planned activities to stabilize.
- Working stage:
  - Identity establishment, beginning to date, sex, drug experimentation, handling money, responsibilities of driving, vocational plans.

© 2014 American Nurses Credentialing Center

Activity Therapy Groups

560

- Types
  - Occupational therapy
  - Recreational therapy
  - Art therapy
  - Drama therapy
  - Dance/Movement therapy
  - Poetry and Bibliotherapy
  - Exercise therapy
- Useful for
  - Psychiatric inpatient and outpatient settings
  - Extended care settings
  - Rehabilitation healthcare settings

© 2014 American Nurses Credentialing Center

Specialized Psychotherapy Groups

561

- Goals
  - Increase personal growth
  - Modify maladaptive behaviors
  - Learn more productive interpersonal responses
  - Develop insights about personal behaviors
- Examples
  - Dialectical Behavioral Therapy (DBT) Groups (developed by Marsha Lineham, PhD)
  - Experiential
  - Focus
  - Encounter
  - Psychodrama
- Useful for clients dealing with varying mental health issues

© 2014 American Nurses Credentialing Center

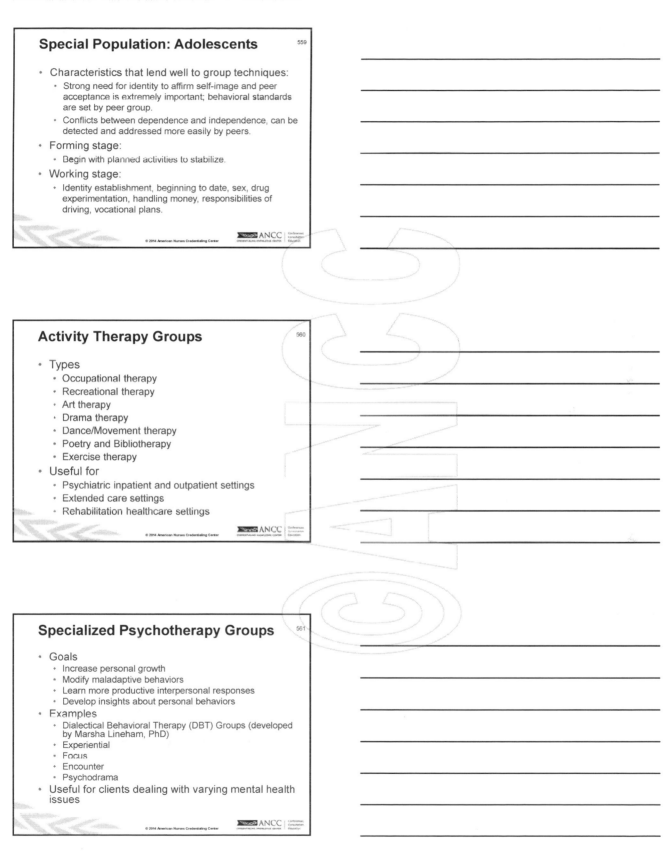

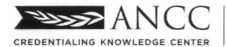
Patient-Family Dimensions

562

- Systems
  - How does one person's mental disorder affect others?
- Gender
  - What are the family roles?
- Developmental
  - What is the family's stage of development?

- Cultural
  - How does the family interact at mealtime, celebrate holidays, etc.
- Conflict
  - How is disagreement between individuals and generations resolved?
- Structural
  - How is nurturing expressed?

© 2014 American Nurses Credentialing Center

Family Structure

563

- Membership categories
  - Nuclear
  - Extended
  - Single-parent
  - Blended
  - Same-sex households
  - Sandwich generation households
  - Polygamy, open marriages/relationships, or cohabitation
- Relationship quality
  - Each with different demands, roles, and expectations
  - Power structure: Who makes decisions?
  - Role structure: Who performs which tasks?

© 2014 American Nurses Credentialing Center

Family Assessment

564

- Risk (susceptibility) factors
  - Substance use
  - Poor family management, parenting, or conflict
  - Poor maternal-child relationships
  - Marital discord
  - History of violence or trauma
  - Physical, sexual, emotional abuse, or neglect
  - Lack of support or weak social ties
  - Poverty/homelessness

- Protective (resilience) factors
  - Cohesion, warmth, or attachment
  - Parental supervision
  - Interaction and communication between and among family
  - Access to healthcare
  - Safe living environments
  - Education
  - Social/community support

© 2014 American Nurses Credentialing Center

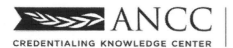
Patient-Family Centered Nursing Care

565

* Family as context
  * Work with patients within the context of family
  * Example: Patient-Family groups pre-discharge
* Family as client
  * Work with the family
  * Example: Marriage and Family Premarital Counseling
* Family as system
  * Work with the family and interconnected systems
  * Example: Nurse-Family Partnership Program
    * An evidence based program that demonstrates better outcomes for new 1st time mothers and their infants

© 2014 American Nurses Credentialing Center

Characteristics of Family Systems

566

* Families
  * Open social systems that interact with many larger systems: Political, religious, school, or health settings.
  * Have a tendency to resist change in order to maintain a steady state of equilibrium.
  * Have goals, structures, roles, and functions.

* Goals vary according to family stage of development, values, and individual concerns.

© 2014 American Nurses Credentialing Center

Family Function/Dysfunction

567

* Function: What family does to achieve goals
  * Clear, open, honest communication enhances problem-solving and conflict resolution, and facilitates coping with life-threatening stressors.
  * Able to nurture and promote growth, parent effectively.
  * Clear and appropriate sexual relationships and boundaries.
* Dysfunction: May result when psychological needs of family members are not met
* Family Genogram: Tool used to assess family structure

© 2014 American Nurses Credentialing Center

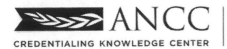
Family Therapy: Purpose and Goals

568

- Purpose
  - Improved interpersonal skills, communication, behavior, and functioning
  - Improved interactions relative to problem behaviors or social systems
  - Enhanced support and nurturing
  - Enhanced internal and external support
  - Adoption of adaptive coping to circumstances
- Goals
  - Individual change or long-term changes in family dynamics
- Techniques
  - Education, support, and skills building

© 2014 American Nurses Credentialing Center

Family Therapy Implementations

569

- Theoretical Frameworks
  - Family systems theory views family as a complex, organized, interactive and holistic organism.
  - Family is a defined group connected by blood or emotional ties with distinct relationship/interaction patterns.
- Two Essential Principles
  - Family is a behavioral system with unique properties, rather than the sum of its part; each part mutually influences and reciprocates the other.
  - Family assumed to be emotionally close and functions interdependently; boundaries differentiate.

© 2014 American Nurses Credentialing Center

Forms of Family Therapy Implementations

570

- Insight-oriented
  - Psychodynamic focus (Murray Bowen)
    - Family of origin: Goal is to foster member differentiation and decrease emotional reactivity and cutoff, triangulation, sibling position, multigenerational transmission process.

© 2014 American Nurses Credentialing Center

Forms of Family Therapy Implementations

571

- Behavioral-oriented
  - Structural focus (Salvador Minuchin)
    - Systems, subsystems, boundaries, "join" family to restructure/reframe.
  - Strategic focus (Jay Haley and Cloe Mandanes)
    - Inequality of power, flawed communication, repetitive and maladaptive family interaction patterns serve a function to control relationships.
  - Solution-focused
    - Pragmatic, short-term, strength-based approach lies with the patient.
  - Multi-Systemic Therapy
    - Evidence-based, family/home-based with adolescents involved with the juvenile justice system.

© 2014 American Nurses Credentialing Center

Family Services: Community-Based

572

- Nurse-Family Partnership:
  - Evidence-based free nurse home visitation program for 1st time moms (pregnancy through age 2).
- Wellness Recovery Action Plan (WRAP)
  - Home and school based individualized intensive mental health services for families with children and adolescents designed to avoid more restrictive placements.

© 2014 American Nurses Credentialing Center

Review Question

573

A female patient, dressed in a sweatshirt and steel-toed boots, tells the nurse that she works as a welder on a construction crew, and her female partner watches their daughter. The nurse understands that this type of androgenous arrangement suggests a:

a) Blended family
b) Disturbed family
c) Same-sex family
d) Sandwich generation family

© 2014 American Nurses Credentialing Center

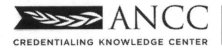

574

People with mental illnesses
enrich our lives

© 2014 American Nurses Credentialing Center

**Advocacy: Deinstitutionalization and
Community Mental Health**

575

- 1960s: Start reduction of state hospitalizations for mentally ill; new focus on community outpatient services.
- Unfortunately, discharges occurred before community programs were sufficient and in place.
- Patients not accustomed to independence were released and urged to mainstream.
  - Patients not prepared with appropriate life skills; many went back to families who were unable to cope.
- Funding inadequate to increase providers in outpatient settings; roles for practitioners changed drastically.
- Transitional and group housing was developed in some areas but not others.

© 2014 American Nurses Credentialing Center

Advocacy: Multi-System Implementations

576

- The integration of therapies and psychopharmacological treatments address a variety of risk factors across the life span (family, peer, school, and community levels).
  - Primary care services required to integrate mental health services in all practices at all specialty levels.
  - Family and community-based treatment to prevent youth out-of-home placements represents the highest level of research evidence of effectiveness for treating youth.
  - Patient Centered Medical Homes are proliferating under the Affordable Care Act.

© 2014 American Nurses Credentialing Center

Advocacy: Organizations 577

- Governmental
  - SAMHSA
  - Centers for Disease Control (CDC)
  - NIH: NIDA, NIMH (The BRAIN Initiative), NCCAM, NINDS
  - U.S. Department of Health and Human Services (USDHHS)
  - U.S. Department of Housing and Urban Development (USHUD)
  - U.S. Department of Agriculture (USDA)
- Not-For-Profit
  - Mental Health Associations
  - National Alliance for Mentally Ill (NAMI)
  - Institute for Healthcare Improvement (IHI)

Surgeon General Report 578

- 1999 groundbreaking report promoted by US Surgeon General David Satcher, MD:
  - *"Americans assign high priority to preventing disease and promoting personal well-being and public health; so, too, must we assign priority to the task of promoting mental health and preventing mental disorders."*
- Disease prevention efforts in mental health are aimed at keeping mental health disorders from appearing, delaying onset, stopping or slowing progression, or minimizing impact on a person's life.

Healthy People 2020: Population Health Promotion Initiatives 579

- Overall goals defined by the US DHHS every 10 years (since 1990) specifies targets with measures.
  - Increase the years and quality of life for all Americans.
  - Reduce current health disparities.
- Initiatives defined across all health domains, including mental health and substance abuse.
- Examples related to mental health/illness:
  - Reduce suicide rate by ____% by year _____.
  - Reduce homelessness in the mentally ill.
  - Increase health screening.
  - Reduce relapse rates.
  - Deliver culturally competent care.

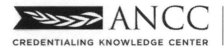
Global Burden of Disease (WHO)

580

- Approximately 14% of the global burden of disease is due to neuropsychiatric disorders (2005). "I had a black dog; his name was depression."
- Burden of depression and other mental health conditions is on the rise globally.
- Suicide: Among top 20 leading causes of death globally for all ages. Annually: Nearly 1 million.
- World Mental Health Day: 10/10 annually
- Human Rights Day: 12/2013: in mental health MINDbank, "Quality Rights" initiative.

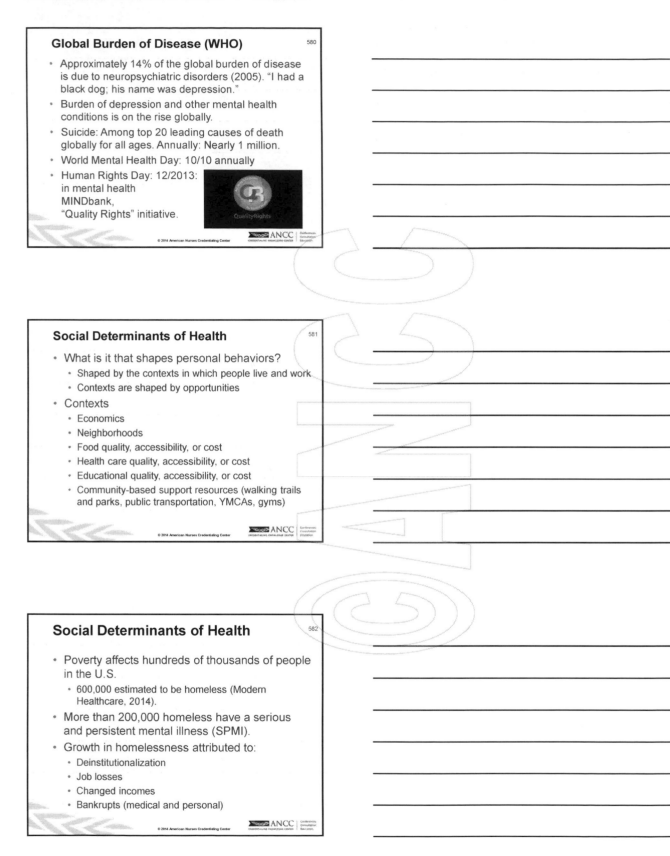

Social Determinants of Health

581

- What is it that shapes personal behaviors?
  - Shaped by the contexts in which people live and work
  - Contexts are shaped by opportunities
- Contexts
  - Economics
  - Neighborhoods
  - Food quality, accessibility, or cost
  - Health care quality, accessibility, or cost
  - Educational quality, accessibility, or cost
  - Community-based support resources (walking trails and parks, public transportation, YMCAs, gyms)

Social Determinants of Health

582

- Poverty affects hundreds of thousands of people in the U.S.
  - 600,000 estimated to be homeless (Modern Healthcare, 2014).
- More than 200,000 homeless have a serious and persistent mental illness (SPMI).
- Growth in homelessness attributed to:
  - Deinstitutionalization
  - Job losses
  - Changed incomes
  - Bankrupts (medical and personal)

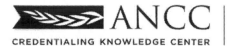

Social Determinants of Health

583

- Homelessness often follows job and welfare losses.
  - Welfare-entitlement system changes have increased the needs of those least able to function.
  - As people come off welfare and hold minimum wage jobs, they often face lack of health insurance and impaired housing.
  - Those most in need become disenfranchised and victimized by the system that pushed them out.
  - Services are often cut first to those with the least voice to protest.
- The fastest growing homeless population are children and youth.

© 2014 American Nurses Credentialing Center

Homelessness and SPMI

584

- SPMI are homeless for longer periods of time; more visible, residing on streets, in parks, subways, and under bridges.
- At least half have a co-occurring substance use disorder.
- SPMI are generally in poorer physical health than other homeless persons.
- Most are eligible for, but few receive, income assistance, including SSI and public assistance.
- Minorities, especially people of color, are overrepresented among the SPMI homeless population.
- Most are willing to accept treatment, but initially are more likely to want help in meeting basic survival needs.

© 2014 American Nurses Credentialing Center

Results of Poverty

585

- Reduced housing options; overcrowded/substandard housing.
- Lack of access to health care.
- Lack of access to quality schools and educational services.
- Dangerous and toxic environments.
- Lack of access to information, technology, and services.
- Decreased likelihood to have access to quality schools.
- Increased levels of crime.
- Greater overall life stress.

© 2014 American Nurses Credentialing Center

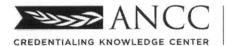

Advocacy: Outreach

586

- Crucial to link SPMI homeless to services (often won't seek treatment on their own).
  - Formerly homeless people are an important resource to engage current homeless.
  - Once involved, provisions made for follow-up case management to meet health, mental health, and social service needs.
  - Needs assessment, and access to appropriate substance abuse treatment is essential.
  - Services must be sensitive to people from diverse cultures, ethnic groups, and special populations (LGBTQI communities).
  - Links to entitlements and opportunities for employment are essential to maintaining residential stability.
- Responses by service providers must consider the individual's perception of need.

© 2014 American Nurses Credentialing Center

Coordination of Care: Standard 5A

587

- Coordination of Care is an implementation.

- Case management is a collaborative process to assess, plan, implement, coordinate, monitor, and evaluate options and services to meet patient health needs through closer communication and connecting to available resources to promote quality cost-effective outcomes.

© 2014 American Nurses Credentialing Center

Advocacy: Case Manager

588

- Coordinates comprehensive health services for continuity of care.
- Accountable for short- and long-range clinical outcomes, as well as overall financial outcomes.
- Partnering with multidisciplinary team ensures that diagnostic and treatment approaches are appropriate and delivered promptly.
- Avoids service duplication and use of unnecessary resources.
- Promotes use of medications on formulary.
- Outpatient programs align discharged patients back to the community as soon as care is coordinated.

© 2014 American Nurses Credentialing Center

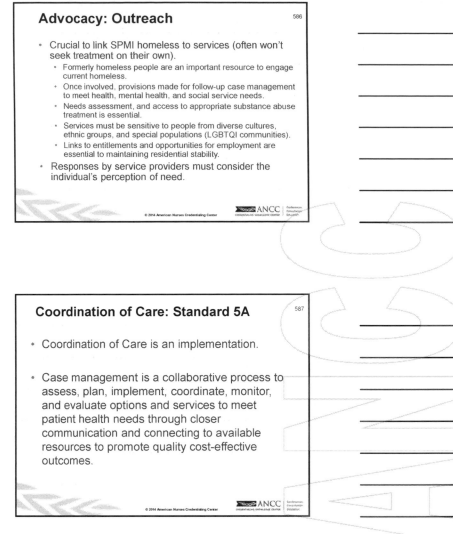

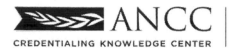
Advocacy: Coordination and Care Models

589

- Mobile Crisis Units/Centers
- Screening, Brief Intervention and Referral to Treatment (SBIRT)
- Assertive Community Treatment Teams (ACCT)
- Homeless shelters
- Community food banks
- Support groups
- Hospice and Respite care
- Transportation assistance
- Long-term care center
- Recovery Model
- Recuperative Care Centers in CA
  - Funded by U.S. Dept. Housing and Urban Development (HUD) partnering with hospitals to provide medical respite.

© 2014 American Nurses Credentialing Center

Advocacy: Public Policy

590

- American with Disabilities Act of 1990
- Mental Health Parity Act of 1996
  - Physical/mental health insurance covered equally
- Drug Addiction Treatment Act of 2000
  - Only ASAM-certified MDs can prescribe buprenorphine
- Paul Wellstone and Pete Domenici Mental Health Parity and Addiction Equity Act of 2008 (final rule 2013)
  - Physical/mental health insurance NOW covered equally
- Protection and Advocacy for Mentally Ill Individuals Act of 2010 (initiated 1986) and Affordable Care Act
  - Expansion of physical/mental health insurance to former uninsured populations
  - Patient Centered Medical Homes

© 2014 American Nurses Credentialing Center

Advocacy: Health Care Systems

591

- Most states: Duty To Warn law
  - Healthcare professional responsible for assessing for threats of violence, identifying the person being threatened, and implementing some affirmative, preventive acts.
- All states have some form of mandatory reporting law for child abuse and neglect.
- Most states have laws for mandatory reporting of elder/vulnerable adult abuse, neglect, or exploitation.
- Most states require reporting of contagious diseases, gunshot wounds, and stabbings.

© 2014 American Nurses Credentialing Center

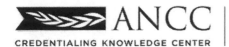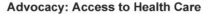

Advocacy: Access to Health Care   592

- Access to Health Care
  - Patient Protection and Affordable Care Act: Everyone afforded health insurance
  - Expansion of Medicare and Medicaid
- Medicaid benefits still only fit a portion of those in need and do not fit most of the poor.
  - Working poor often make too much money for entitlements.
- Many agencies are denying treatment to those unable to pay up front.

© 2014 American Nurses Credentialing Center

Advocacy: Recovery Model for Mental Health Treatment Outcomes   593

Recovery is… "…both a conceptual framework for understanding mental illness and a system of care to provide supports and opportunities for personal development. Recovery emphasizes that while individuals may not be able to have full control over their symptoms, they can have full control over their lives. Recovery asserts that persons with psychiatric disabilities can achieve not only affective stability and social rehabilitation, but transcend limits imposed by both mental illness and social barriers to achieve their highest goals and aspirations."

The Recovery Model, Contra Costa County, CA

© 2014 American Nurses Credentialing Center

Patient is the Teacher; Nurse the Pupil   594

- Recovery
  - Is possible even from SPMI,
  - May be difficult;
  - Differs among people;
  - Is holistic;
  - Promotes self-determination, self-advocacy, hope, and empowerment;
  - Is facilitated through peer and systems supports and programs;
  - Focuses on strengths and resilience, not just disabilities; and
  - Focuses on personalized support systems, not just clinical symptoms.

© 2014 American Nurses Credentialing Center

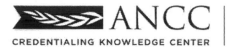
Advocacy: Psychiatric Mental Health Nurse

595

- Purpose
  - Promote pro-health patient and family-centered care.
- Ways to advocate
  - Work toward changing legislation; stay abreast of politics.
  - Legislate for mental health and substance abuse funding.
  - Empower patients/others to speak up.
  - Challenge non-supportive systems.
  - Sponsor/participate in pro-mental health events (e.g., Out of Darkness walks; Suicide Hotlines, Mental Health Events; World Suicide Prevention Day, National Alliance for Mental Illness Walks).
  - Provide community education to reduce stigma, discrimination, and criminalization.
  - Challenge stigmatizing and discriminatory language descriptions. (crazy, psycho, lunatic, borderline, etc.).
- Other examples
  - Tobacco-Free Nurses; Sexual Assault Nurse Examiners (SANE) education and preparation.

© 2014 American Nurses Credentialing Center

Advocacy: Attitudes

596

- Stigma, discrimination, and criminalization
  - Although thought to be more violent, and often treated as though they are violent, people with mental illnesses are no more violent than those in the average population.
  - If there is no diagnosis of substance use disorder, they are no more violent than persons without mental illnesses. Substance use, however, increases the risk for violence among those with mental illnesses.
- Violence risk is increased in a person with a mental illness who is experiencing control hallucinations and is not medicated.
- With current problems accessing health care, there will be more violence problems exhibited.

© 2014 American Nurses Credentialing Center

Advocacy: Attitudes

597

- Language considerations – eliminating terms like:
  - "Alcoholic" or "drug addict" or "junkie" instead, person with a substance abuse problem,
  - "Crazy" or "psycho" or "lunatic" instead, person with a mental illness.

© 2014 American Nurses Credentialing Center

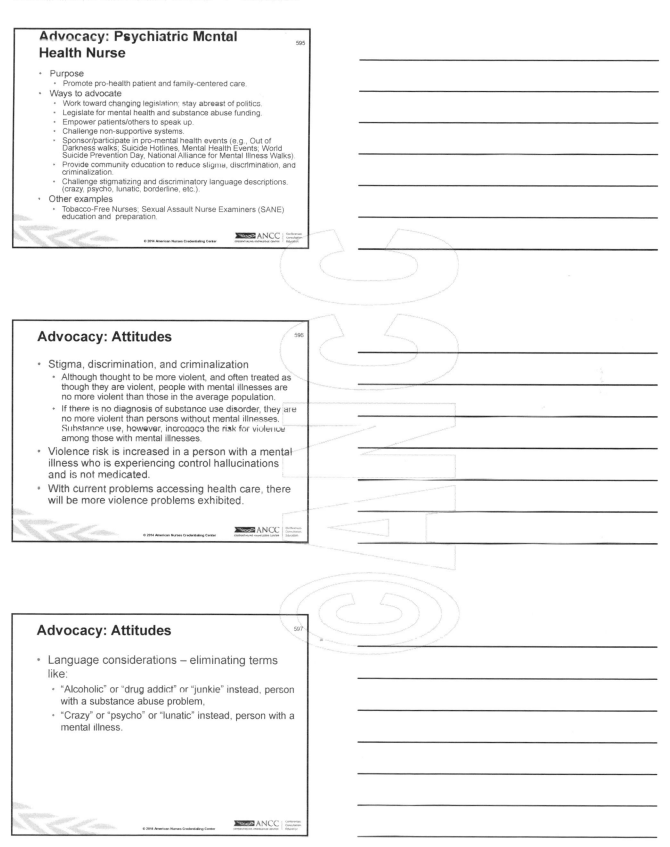

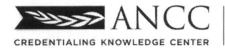
Optimizing Treatment Effectiveness

598

- In general, psychotropic medications in combination with therapy (particularly CBT) produce better treatment results and remission rates.

- Advocacy, public policy, and community supports are designed to reduce recidivism and promote overall health and wellness.

- "Health is a state of complete physical, mental, and social well-being and not merely the absence of disease or infirmity" (World Health Organization).

© 2014 American Nurses Credentialing Center

Review Question

599

14-year old Anna is being seen at the community health clinic after referral from the local school health nurse. Anna has no stable family life; social history reveals that she is in and out of foster care homes. Classmates had reported, "Anna had not been going to classes or doing anything with us for 2 weeks. She's been crying in the bathroom a lot". It was learned that Anna participated in a weekend binge drinking splurge in which she woke up alone in a fraternity hall with her panties askew. At the initial assessment, Anna is voicing vague recollections of feeling pressured by older guys and girls. What services are appropriate for Anna?

a) Examination by SANE or designee, consult with social services.
b) Education about safe sex practices and assertiveness training.
c) Neuropsychiatric testing, urine drug screen.
d) Referral for STI consult, case management, and social services.
e) Consultation with chaplain or designee, support with notifying authorities about the fraternity infractions.

© 2014 American Nurses Credentialing Center

Review Question

600

- The patient with borderline personality disorder informs the nurse that she "keeps losing boyfriends. They always leave me after I have given them my life. How can I be fixed? What is wrong with me?" What statement by the nurse is appropriate for this patient?

a) "Once you work with dialectical behavior therapies, you may gain an understanding as to how you are communicating with others."
b) After six weeks of daily regulation with citalopram (Celexa) 40 mg, you will not see this issue as totally your fault."
c) "Your problem stems from early childhood abandonment. You will have to learn to accept people for what they are, and not what you think they should be."
d) "Cognitive behavioral therapy works by helping you refute this negative thinking and uplift your self esteem."

© 2014 American Nurses Credentialing Center

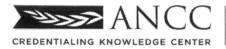

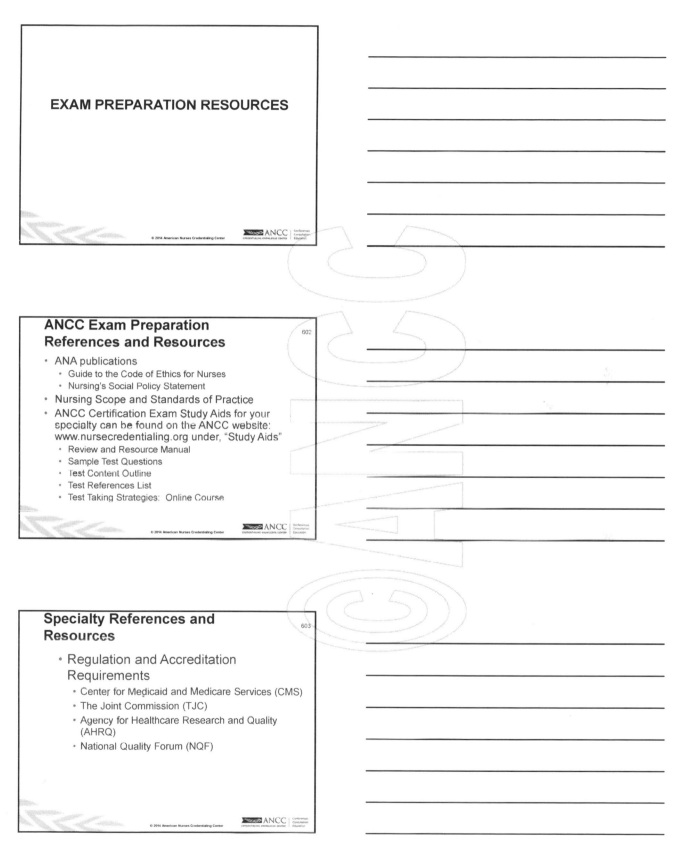

EXAM PREPARATION RESOURCES

© 2014 American Nurses Credentialing Center

ANCC Exam Preparation References and Resources

602

- ANA publications
  - Guide to the Code of Ethics for Nurses
  - Nursing's Social Policy Statement
- Nursing Scope and Standards of Practice
- ANCC Certification Exam Study Aids for your specialty can be found on the ANCC website: www.nursecredentialing.org under, "Study Aids"
  - Review and Resource Manual
  - Sample Test Questions
  - Test Content Outline
  - Test References List
  - Test Taking Strategies: Online Course

© 2014 American Nurses Credentialing Center

Specialty References and Resources

603

- Regulation and Accreditation Requirements
  - Center for Medicaid and Medicare Services (CMS)
  - The Joint Commission (TJC)
  - Agency for Healthcare Research and Quality (AHRQ)
  - National Quality Forum (NQF)

© 2014 American Nurses Credentialing Center

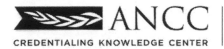

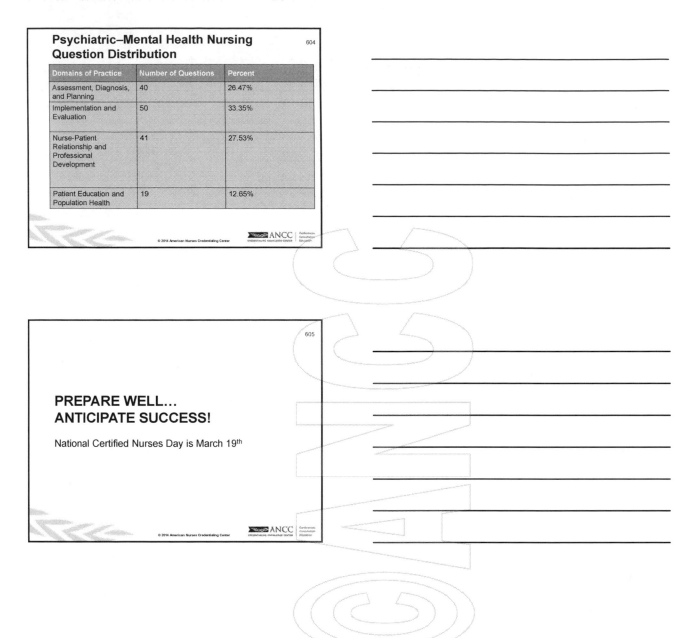

Psychiatric–Mental Health Nursing Question Distribution

604

Domains of Practice	Number of Questions	Percent
Assessment, Diagnosis, and Planning	40	26.47%
Implementation and Evaluation	50	33.35%
Nurse-Patient Relationship and Professional Development	41	27.53%
Patient Education and Population Health	19	12.65%

© 2014 American Nurses Credentialing Center

605

PREPARE WELL…
ANTICIPATE SUCCESS!

National Certified Nurses Day is March 19th

© 2014 American Nurses Credentialing Center

References

American Nurses Association. *Guide to the Code of Ethics for Nurses: Interpretation and Application.* Silver Spring, MD: Nursesbooks.org; 2008.

American Nurses Association. *Nursing: Scope and Standards of Practice*. 2nd ed. Silver Spring, MD: Nursesbooks.org; 2010.

American Psychiatric Association. *Diagnostic and Statistical Manual of Mental Disorders (DSM-5)*. 5th ed. Arlington, VA: American Psychiatric Publishing; 2013.

American Psychiatric Nurses Association, International Society of Psychiatric- Mental Health Nurses, American Nurses Association. *Psychiatric-Mental Health Nursing: Scope and Standards of Practice*. Silver Spring, MD: Nursesbooks.org; 2007.

Andrews MM, Boycle JS. *Transcultural Concepts in Nursing Care.* 6th ed. Philadelphia, PA: Lippincott Williams & Wilkins; 2012.

Antai-Otong D. *Psychiatric Nursing: Biological & Behavioral Concepts*. 2nd ed. New York, NY: CengageBrain.com (Cengage Learning); 2008.

Boyd MA. *Psychiatric Nursing: Contemporary Practice*. 5th ed. Philadelphia, PA: Lippincott Williams & Wilkins; 2012.

Jarvis C, ed. *Physical Examination and Health Assessment*. 6th ed. St Louis, MO: Saunders; 2012.

Lipson JG, Dibble SL, eds. *Culture and Clinical Care*. 2nd ed. San Francisco, CA: UCSF Nursing Press; 2005.

Marriner Tomey A. *Guide to Nursing Management and Leadership*. 8th ed. St Louis, MO: Mosby Inc.; 2009.

Polit DF, Beck CT. *Nursing Research: Generating and Assessing Evidence for Nursing Practice*. 9th ed. Philadelphia, PA: Lippincott Williams & Wilkins; 2011.

Skidmore-Roth L. *Mosby's 2014 Nursing Drug Reference*. 27th ed. St Louis, MO: Mosby Inc; 2014.

Varcarolis EM, Halter MJ. *Foundations of Psychiatric Mental Health Nursing: A Clinical Approach*. 6th ed. Philadelphia, PA: Saunders; 2010.

Additional References

AHRQ: Tobacco 5 A's:
https://www.ahrq.gov/professionals/clinicians-providers/guidelines-recommendations/tobacco/5steps.html

Crettol J, de Leon J, Hiemke C and Eap CB. (March 2014). "Pharmacogenomics in Psychiatry:From Therapeutic Drug Monitoring to Genomic Medicine". Nature, Vol 95(3), pp 254-257.

Dolgin E. (April 2014). Negative Feedback. Nature, Vol 508; pp S10-S11.

Farrington, E. "Relationship of Vitamin D Deficiency to Depression in Older Adults: An Integrative Review for 2008-2013". Faculty Advisor: Mary Moller, Yale School of Nursing. Poster presented at 27th Annual APNA Conference 2013.

Healthy People Initiative:
www.cdc.gov/nchs/healthy_people/hp2020/hp2020_progress_reviews.htm

http://www.cdc.gov/nchs/ppt/hp2020/hp2020_MH_MD_and_SA_progress_review_presentation.pdf

MINT: Excellence in motivational interviewing: http://www.motivationalinterviewing.org/

Multimodal Therapy: http://en.wikipedia.org/wiki/Multimodal_therapy

NANDA-I sources:
http://www.nanda.org/
http://kb.nanda.org/article/AA-00233/34/English-/Frequently-Asked-Questions/About-NANDA-International/What-does-NANDA-stand-for.html

http://faculty.mu.edu.sa/public/uploads/1380604673.6151NANDA%202012.pdf

http://nclex.ucoz.net/_ld/0/30_NANDALISTOFDIAG.pdf

Nihilistic delusions video: https://www.youtube.com/watch?v=zX9OTDzyNdQ

NIMH Website for information and images for: electroconvulsant therapy (ECT), transmagnetic stimulation therapy (TMS), vagal nerve stimulation (VNS), and deep brain stimulation (DBS):
http://www.nimh.nih.gov/health/topics/brain-stimulation-therapies/brain-stimulation-therapies.shtml

Owen DC, Armstrong ML, Koch JR, and Roberts AE. (October 2013). College students with body art. J psychosocial nursing, 51(10), 20-28.

Patient's Bill of Rights (CMS, 2010)
http://www.cms.gov/CCIIO/Programs-and-Initiatives/Health-Insurance-Market-Reforms/Patients-Bill-of-Rights.html

Rett Syndrome: http://www.ninds.nih.gov/disorders/rett/detail_rett.htm

Schizophrenia video from Nature pub April 2014:
http://www.nature.com/nature/outlook/schizophrenia/#video

Substance Abuse and Mental Illness Are Linked.
http://www.cdc.gov/nchs/ppt/hp2020/hp2020_MH_MD_and_SA_progress_review_presentation.pdf

USDHHS Family History Initiative: http://www.hhs.gov/familyhistory/

World Health Organization: Burden of Global Disease:
http://www.who.int/mental_health/en/

http://www.who.int/mediacentre/factsheets/fs369/en/

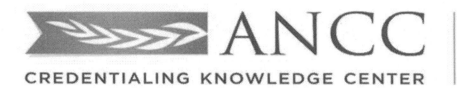

Psychiatric-Mental Health Nursing Appendices

I-Test Taking Strategies

II-Test Content Outline

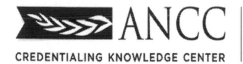

CREDENTIALING KNOWLEDGE CENTER

Conferences.
Consultation.
Education.

Taking the Certification Exam

Test Taking Tips and Strategies

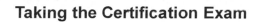

Taking the Certification Exam
Test Taking Tips & Strategies

- Why Certify?
  - Validates specialty knowledge
  - Reflects commitment to the profession of nursing
  - Demonstrates accountability to the public at large

© 2014 American Nurses Credentialing Center

Review Course

- Supplements your individual knowledge
- Provides a brief review of test content
- Helps build self-confidence that you CAN pass the exam
- Prepares you well so you can anticipate success

© 2014 American Nurses Credentialing Center

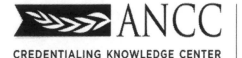

Gather Personal Resources

- Current texts
- ANCC review manuals
- ANA publications
  - Guide to the Code of Ethics for Nurses
  - Nursing's Social Policy Statement
- Standards for your practice discipline
- Professional journals
- Web sites

Include a Review of Web References for Your Specialty

- Standards and references are available on the Internet that apply to your specialty
  - Review Healthy People 2020 Focus Areas
  - CDC Immunization guidelines

- ANCC Web site: practice questions and Test Content Outline
  - www.nursecredentialing.org

Information Materials from ANCC

- Review and refer to materials frequently to gain insight into test content and sample questions

- Review the Test Content Outline and be clear about the percentage of questions in each section of the test

- Keep entry letter to exam in a safe place and bring it with you to the exam; this is not a form of I.D.

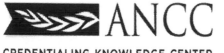

General Suggestions for Test Preparation

- Study over time for maximum effectiveness
- Set reasonable expectations
  - Do not expect to know everything—you do not need a perfect score to pass the test
  - What do you need to know? Print out Test Content Outline as a guide
  - Learn the general rules, not the exceptions
  - Exam is designed to be at a moderate experience level

More Suggestions for Test Preparation

- Review references for your specialty certification exam found on the ANCC Web site
- Do not listen to gossip about the exam, computerized test bank delivers random questions in topics defined in the Test Content Outline
- Prepare mentally and physically
- Practice with sample questions

Know Your Test Taking Style

- Do not rush through exam—pace yourself
- Read directions and questions carefully
- Do not dwell on one question for a long time
- Spend an average of 45 to 60 seconds per question and move on, return at end to review answers you were unsure of
- Answer easier questions first

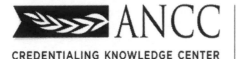
Institute a Study Plan

10

- Set a schedule and stick to it
- If you procrastinate get help from a friend or reorganize your plan
- Know the basic content knowledge and be able to use this information critically to think and make decisions about facts
- Memorize the basics

Personalize Your Study Plan

11

- Allow for breaks as you study
- Adjust plan according to your learning needs
- Using your study guide from the review, identify strong and weak areas
- Review FIRST what you know LEAST
- Look for key words
- Review and practice sample questions
- Prepare to answer ONLY what is asked

Prepare for Question Format

12

- Analyze the question carefully
  - Look for key words or phrases that lead you
- Read all the answers first
  - Many questions do not have one right answer, be sure you answer the question asked
- Multiple choice questions

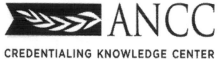
Specific Test Taking Skills

13

- For multiple choice questions, eliminate answers you know are not correct
- In a question with an "all of the above" choice, if you see at least two correct statements, then "all of the above" is most likely the correct answer
- Answers that are more positive are more likely to be correct than negative ones
- Answers that are more informative are more likely to be correct

© 2014 American Nurses Credentialing Center

Specific Test Taking Skills

14

- Avoid changing answers
- Time yourself to complete the whole exam
  - There is no penalty for a wrong answer
  - Do not leave blanks
- Review your work if time allows

© 2014 American Nurses Credentialing Center

The Night Before the Exam

15

- Plan to arrive early, know directions to the testing center, how long it will take to get to the exam, park, and get to room assigned

- If possible, do a test run to the testing site the night before to determine travel time, primary route and alternate route, parking, and exact location of the testing center
  - The test run to the testing site can help to decrease stress

- Don't try to pull an all-nighter, get a good night's sleep before the exam
  - Cramming and lack of sleep will affect performance

© 2014 American Nurses Credentialing Center

© 2014 American Nurses Credentialing Center.

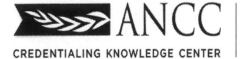

The Night Before the Exam

- Eat before the exam
  - Having food in your stomach will give you energy and help you focus
  - Avoid heavy foods which can make you groggy

- Avoid foods laden with sugar

- Eat sensibly to aid concentration and minimize fatigue

- Avoid alcohol and anxiety/sedative medication

Know Your Testing Center: Regulations and Identification

- Prior to the day of the exam:
  - Review testing center Web site for specific testing center regulations
- On the day of the exam:
  - You will be required to provide valid (unexpired) and acceptable forms of identification upon arrival at the testing center
  - Validity and number of ID's required is predetermined by your test sponsor
  - Examples of identification:
    - Driver's license
    - State identification
    - Passport
    - U.S. military identification

More Information on Identification

- Identification must:
  - Be valid (unexpired)
  - Contain BOTH your signature and recent (no more than 10 years old) photograph
  - Be in English and signed in English

- The ANCC confirmation letter is not an acceptable form of I.D.

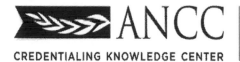
Know Your Testing Center: Testing Center Regulations

19

- Please review the testing center Web site for additional testing center regulations

- Regulations include important information on test monitoring, communication, items permitted in the testing room, and general security items

© 2014 American Nurses Credentialing Center

Know Your Testing Center: Personal/Unauthorized Items

20

- You will not be permitted to bring any personal/unauthorized items into the testing room and will be required to lock up all personal items before entering the testing area

- Examples of personal/unauthorized items include:
  - Books, paper, calculators, Kleenex, food*, drink*, water*, notes, watches, cell phones, PDA, personal electronics* of any kind

© 2014 American Nurses Credentialing Center

Dressing and Thoughts for Success

21

- Wear comfortable clothing
- Bright colors, especially reds and yellows are invigorating
  - Colors are neither good or bad but they influence the human psyche
- Looking good = feeling good
- Don't panic—deep breaths help relieve stress
- Ignore others who finish early
- Use all of the time allotted if you require it

Prepare well and anticipate success!

© 2014 American Nurses Credentialing Center

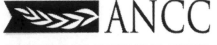
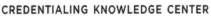

References

22

- Hemphill, M. (1996). A note on adults color-emotion association. The Journal of Genetic Psychology, 157(3), 275-280.

- Kantrowitz, M. (nd). Top Standardized Test-taking Tips. Retrieved from http://www.fastweb.com/college-search/articles/1707-top standardized-test-taking-tips.

- Ten Tips for Terrific Test Taking. Retrieved from http://www.studygs.net/tsttak1.htm.

© 2014 American Nurses Credentialing Center

_____

_____

_____

_____

_____

_____

_____

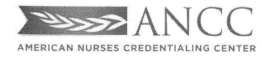

8515 Georgia Ave, Suite 400   1.800.284.2378

Silver Spring, MD 20910   nursecredentialing.org

Test Content Outline
Effective Date: October 25, 2014

Psychiatric and Mental Health Nursing
Board Certification Examination

There are 175 questions on this examination. Of these, 150 are scored questions and 25 are pretest questions that are not scored. Pretest questions are used to determine how well these questions will perform before they are used on the scored portion of the examination. The pretest questions cannot be distinguished from those that will be scored, so it is important for a candidate to answer all questions. A candidate's score, however, is based solely on the 150 scored questions. Performance on pretest questions does not affect a candidate's score.

This Test Content Outline identifies the areas that are included on the examination. The percentage and number of questions in each of the major categories of the scored portion of the examination are also shown.

Category	Domains of Practice	No. of Questions	Percent
I	Assessment, Diagnosis, and Planning	40	26.47%
II	Implementation and Evaluation	50	33.35%
III	Nurse-Patient Relationship and Professional Development	41	27.53%
IV	Patient Education and Population Health	19	12.65%
	Total	150	100%

I. Assessment, Diagnosis and Planning (26%)

A. Assessment
   Knowledge of:

1. Assessment tools and techniques (e.g., Mini–Mental State Examination [MMSE], patient history, functional status, developmental milestones, clinical interview)
2. Developmental stages (e.g. Maslow, Erickson, Piaget)

   Skill in:

3. Obtaining patient history using age-appropriate, system-specific, standardized/evidence-based tools
4. Obtaining a current medication and treatment list
5. Assessing for use of complementary and alternative methods (e.g., therapeutic touch, herbal preparations, acupuncture)
6. Performing a physical assessment using age-appropriate, system-specific, evidence-based tools and techniques
7. Performing a psychosocial assessment using age-appropriate, system-specific, evidence-based tools and techniques
8. Obtaining diagnostic test results
9. Reviewing findings provided by interdisciplinary team and external resources

B. Problem Identification/Nursing Diagnoses
   Knowledge of:

1. Pathophysiology related to mental illness (e.g. normal/abnormal mental changes across the lifespan, altered mental status related to urinary tract infection [UTI], depressive or anxiety disorders related to thyroid dysfunctions)
2. Psychiatric disorders (e.g. schizophrenia spectrum and other psychotic disorders, bipolar and related disorders, substance related and addictive disorders, neurodevelopmental disorders, eating and feeding disorders, personality disorders, disruptive, impulse-control, conduct disorders, anxiety disorder, trauma stress or related)

   Skill in:

3. Identifying nursing diagnoses using a standardized classification system.
4. Identifying barriers to effective communication (e.g., psychosocial, literacy, financial, cultural) and making appropriate adaptations
5. Identifying patterns and variances that pose actual or potential risks to health and safety (e.g., self-harm, abuse, neglect, interpersonal, environmental, lack of external resources) by synthesizing available data and knowledge

C. Planning and Outcomes Identification
   Knowledge of:

1. Plan of care strategies (e.g. interdisciplinary care coordination, health promotion, disease management, symptom reduction)
2. Evidence-based guidelines (e.g. suicide prevention, recovery model)

2

Skill in:

3. Prioritizing nursing diagnoses and/or problems.
4. Formulating expected outcomes with the patient, family, significant other, and interdisciplinary team to facilitate continuity across the continuum of care
5. Developing an individualized, patient-centered age and developmentally appropriate plan of care and expected outcomes

II. Implementation and Evaluation (33%)

A. Implementation
Knowledge of:

1. Psychopharmacology (e.g. indications, allergies, reactions, adverse and contraindications)
2. Complementary and alternative methods (e.g. relaxation, sensory stimulation, guided imagery, aromatherapy)
3. Management of emergent and crisis situations
4. Patient safety and risk reduction interventions, technologies and equipment (e.g. falls, suicide, QT interval monitoring, de-escalations, restraints, assault, behavior management, close observation, video monitoring, alarms)

Skill in:

5. Creating a safe, therapeutic, and developmentally appropriate environment conducive to care (e.g. establishing trust, building rapport, individual factors, milieu management)
6. Implementing age and developmentally appropriate evidence-based nursing interventions specific to the plan of care (e.g. behavior modification, relaxation, coping skills, safety management, group therapy)
7. Collaborating with the interdisciplinary team and external resources to coordinate the plan of care across the continuum
8. Reconciling medications and treatments across transitions of care
9. Administering medications and other treatments that are appropriate to the patient situation
10. Responding proactively to changes in patient condition to prevent or minimize adverse patient outcomes

B. Evaluation
Knowledge of:

1. Expected and unexpected responses to interventions

Skill in:

2. Evaluating patient's response to interventions and effectiveness of the interdisciplinary plan of care
3. Modifying the plan of care in collaboration with patient, family, significant other, and interdisciplinary team based on ongoing assessment data including impact of patient resources (e.g. financial, family, culture and access to community resources)
4. Interpreting patterns and variances related to response to interventions

3

III. Nurse-Patient Relationship and Professional Development (28%)

A. Nurse Patient Relationship
Knowledge of

1. Cultural, religious, and socio-economic factors, family dynamics, and health practices of diverse groups.
2. Developmental response to illness and hospitalization
3. Coping and defense mechanisms (e.g. rationalization, denial, projection, compensation)
4. Care system supports (e.g., respite care, volunteers, transportation, group-specific supports, adult day care, topic specific support group)

Skill in

5. Using therapeutic communication (e.g. active listening, reflection, clarifying, summarizing), with awareness of Verbal / Non-Verbal / Para-Verbal (e.g. tone, cadence, rate) aspects, that are age, developmentally, and situationally appropriate
6. Maintaining appropriate physical and emotional boundaries
7. Developing a therapeutic relationship specific to the patient condition with an awareness of transference and counter-transference dynamics
8. Advocating for the patient by supporting patient's rights and identified support-systems consistent with patient/guardian preference

B. Professional Development
Knowledge of:

1. Current trends (e.g., research, technology, legislative, policy)
2. Professional Organizations (e.g. American Nurses Association [ANA], American Nurses Credentialing Center [ANCC], American Psychiatric Nurses Association [APNA] , International Society of Psychiatric- Mental Health Nurses [ISPN], National Alliance on Mental Illness [NAMI], Substance Abuse and Mental Health Services Administration [SAMHSA] and Activities
3. Documentation Skills (e.g. legal, reimbursement, clinical implications)

Skill in:

4. Delegating elements of care to licensed and/or unlicensed personnel in accordance with applicable legal or policy parameters or principles
5. Identifying and addressing personal attitudes, values, and beliefs in self and others that may negatively impact delivery of care
6. Identifying quality improvement or risk management opportunities (e.g. quality variances, serious reportable events, infectious diseases)

C. C. Leadership
Knowledge of:

1. Legal, regulatory, and ethical considerations (e.g., American Nurses Association [ANA] *Code of Ethics*, influencing healthcare policy, informed consent, Health Insurance Portability and Accountability Act [HIPAA], advance directives, American Disability Act, restraints)

Skill in:

2. Using professional communication (e.g., interdisciplinary communication, conflict resolution, peer review)

4

3. Promoting teamwork and engagement of healthcare providers to manage change and optimize patient care
4. Serving as a clinical resource (e.g., mentor, preceptor, educator) for the advancement of nursing practice, the profession, and quality health care
5. Creating a healthy work environment (e.g., professional boundaries, employee relationships, workplace civility, team building, diversity, shared governance)
6. Coordinating patient safety initiatives

IV. Patient Education and Population Health (13%)

A. Patient Education
Knowledge of:

1. Principles, methods, and concepts of teaching and learning (e.g., motivation/readiness to learn, use of technology, age and developmentally appropriate techniques) for groups and individuals

Skill in:

2. Identifying and prioritizing learning needs (e.g., health literacy, patient expectations and preferences)
3. Adapting for factors that may influence learning (e.g., sensory impairment, cognitive deficits, environment, cultural differences)
4. Developing an individualized education plan that promotes health, wellness, and self-management (e.g., medication management, crisis safety plan, relapse prevention, community resources), with the involvement of the patient, family, and interdisciplinary team
5. Creating an environment conducive to teaching/learning

B. Population Health
Knowledge of:

1. Health promotion strategies (e.g., screenings, immunization, exercise, nutrition, tobacco cessation, drug and alcohol prevention)

Skill in:

2. Developing educational programs for groups and individuals, considering risk behaviors or factors(e.g., substance abuse, homelessness, lack of access to resources, support, and care, medication non-adherence, lifestyles, medical co-morbidities, trauma)
3. Identifying community resources (e.g. homeless shelters, food banks, crisis centers, support groups, hospice) that assist and support patients in self-management

Last Updated 10/11/2013

5

Made in the USA
San Bernardino, CA
14 March 2016